Healing Brain Injury Naturally

written by
Douglas S. Wingate

www.healingbraininjurynaturally.com

Healing Brain Injury Naturally
Douglas S. Wingate
www.healingbraininjurynaturally.com

Note to the Reader: This book is intended as an informational guide and resource. The remedies, approaches, and techniques described herein are meant to supplement, and not be a substitute for, professional medical care or treatment. They should not be used to treat a serious ailment without prior consultation with a qualified health care professional.

The information contained in this book has been compile from sources deemed reliable, and it is accurate to the best of the Author's knowledge; however, the Author cannot guarantee its accuracy and validity and cannot be held liable for any errors or omissions. You must consult your doctor or gt professional medical advice before using any of the suggested remedies, techniques, or information in this book.

Upon using the information contained in this book, you agree to hold harmless the Author from and against any damages, costs, and expenses, including any legal fees potentially resulting from the application of any of the information provided in this guide. This disclaimer applies to any damages or injury caused by the use and application, whether directly or indirectly, of any advice or information presented, whether for breach of contract, tort, negligence, personal injury, criminal intent, or under any other cause of action.

You agree to accept all risks of using the information presented inside this book. You need to consult a professional medical practitioner in order to ensure you are both able and healthy enough to participate in this program or anything within.

TABLE OF CONTENTS

Dedicated to my mother Jeanette Wingate.
Thank you for always being an unending source of love and support

Part 1

Understanding A Brain Injury

Chapter 1
The "Silent Epidemic"

First, some definitions...

Brain injuries that are not congenital, hereditary, degenerative or due to birth trauma are collectively referred to as an "acquired brain injury" (ABI) and are the result of changes in neuronal activity that affect physical integrity, metabolic activity, or functional ability of the nerve cells of the brain. They can occur for a number of different reasons. An acquired brain injury can be placed into two general categories – traumatic and non-traumatic. Much of the information in this book applies to both, though it is primarily directed at traumatic brain injury (TBI) which is defined as being caused by an external force. Direct impact injuries can be further divided into either closed injuries, where there is direct tissue injury or bleeding within the skull, or open injuries, where the skull or surrounding tissue has actually been breached.

ABI = "acquired brain injury": changes in neuronal activity that affect physical integrity, metabolic activity, or functional ability of the nerve cells of the brain

TBI = "traumatic brain injury": an injury to the brain stemming from an external force

Causes of Traumatic Brain Injury	Causes of Non-Traumatic Brain Injury
-Falls -Assaults -Motor vehicle accidents -Sports and recreational injuries -Abusive head trauma/"shaken baby syndrome" -Gunshot wounds -Workplace injuries -Child abuse -Domestic violence -Military actions/blast injuries	-Stroke -Infectious disease (meningitis, encephalitis) -Seizure disorders -Electric shock/lightning strike -Tumors (surgery/radiation/chemo) -Toxic exposures (substance misuse, lead ingestion, inhalation of volatile agents) -Metabolic disorders (insulin shock, diabetic coma, liver and kidney disease) -Neurotoxic poisoning (carbon monoxide, inhalants, lead exposure) -Lack of oxygen to the brain (near drowning, airway obstruction, strangulation, cardiopulmonary arrest, hypoxia, anoxia)

"Sports-related TBI" = distinguished from other causes of TBI, this is a term for brain injuries that occur specifically as a result of a sports injury.

CTE = "chronic traumatic encephalopathy": a rare, progressively degenerative condition of the central nervous system which typically follows repetitive brain trauma

Disability from a brain injury can result both from the primary injury (the initial injury itself), and from secondary injuries sustained over time.

Secondary injuries can stem from lack of oxygen (hypoxia), lack of blood (anemia), excessive fluid in the brain cavity (hydrocephalus), metabolic abnormalities, elevated blood pressure in the skull (intracranial hypertension), and bleeding (hemorrhagic activity). Other factors can also be delayed as a result of injury including the release of excitatory amino acids, free radical production, arachidonic acid metabolite releases and disruptions in neurotransmitters such as serotonin and monoamines.

It is important to keep in mind that *a traumatic brain injury is much more than a single event; it is also not a final outcome.*

Rather, it is often the beginning of a chronic, potentially progressive, process. The injury may impact multiple organ systems and can both cause and accelerate other health problems in the body. In some cases accelerated brain deterioration in the white matter of the frontal and temporal lobes has been found. This may be the result of a defect in regular programmed cell death (apoptosis) causing the cells to not turn over as efficiently as they should. There is evidence that sustaining a TBI may impact recovery rates from future injuries.

It is for all of these reasons that it remains very important for the individual and their healthcare providers to be attentive and vigilant in restoring and maintaining the physical, mental, and emotional state of the individual.

The numbers...

Over 2 million people in the United States sustain a brain injury every year. Over 5.4 million people are living with residual effects of their injury each day. It remains among the leading causes of death and long-term disability. These numbers are made even more staggering when you consider that the incidences of mild brain injury (mTBI) are generally considered to be greatly underreported, so in actuality, many more are occurring.

For these reasons, and the relative lack of attention and discussion given to the topic, brain injury has often been referred to as a "silent epidemic". A brain injury can be difficult to understand if someone has not been directly impacted by one or been close to someone who has. The external initial wounds seemingly heal, while the internal wounds can remain and continue on for years, and sometimes, a lifetime.

A brain injury can result in a wide range of emotional, behavioral and/or cognitive symptoms. These can include a quickness to anger, loss of executive function (discussed later), depression, fatigue, excessive emotionality, socially inappropriate behaviors, or a seeming loss of one's filter when it comes to actions and language (impaired impulse control). If another person is not aware that someone has this kind of injury these can cause great difficulties in social and professional situations. There may appear to be nothing physically "wrong" from an outsiders perspective and they assume no injury exists. Understanding that someone can be impacted by long-standing symptoms that are often very frustrating for the individual can be difficult. For this same reason, those with a brain injury have also been referred to as the "walking wounded". Over time, these difficulties take their toll; not only on the affected person, but stress is placed on on their families, friends, caregivers and social structures. Work, school, and recreational activities can all become affected.

Demographics

Children and Teens
Children ages 0-4 years old have the highest rate of emergency room visits, hospitalizations and deaths combined when it comes to traumatic brain injury. These primarily result from falls, accidents, or abuse. Abusive head trauma, formally called "shaken baby syndrome", is a leading cause of death from brain injury in infants and young children. This is followed by adolescents and young adults ages 15-19 years old who tend to sustain injuries from motor vehicle accidents, falls, and sports injuries. An estimated 1.6 million-3.8 million sports related head injuries happen each year, including those where no medical care is sought. It is estimated that by the age of 25, 38% of males and 24% of females will have experienced at least one incidence of mild to severe brain trauma.

Causes
Overall, falls have been found to be the leading cause of a traumatic brain injury (35.2%), followed by motor vehicle accidents (17.3%), being "struck by/against" (16.5%), and assaults (10%). At least 156,000 TBI-related deaths, hospitalizations, and emergency room visits happen each year as the result of assault. In the United States women experience about 4.8 million intimate partner-related physical assaults annually making the potential number of actual occurrences (including those where no medical attention is sought) significantly higher.

Military Personnel
Military service members are a high risk group with at least 325,000 returning US troops estimated to have some form of a brain injury with or without concomitant post-traumatic stress disorder. According to the Department of Defense website in 2000 there were 10,963 TBI diagnoses. This increased substantially from 2006-2009 in which there averaged 24,074 diagnoses each year, with an estimated 11.2%-22.8% of deployed service members reporting a possible concussion or brain injury.

Economic Impact
The costs of these incidences add up quickly as well – mentally, emotionally, spiritually, and certainly, economically. The total lifetime comprehensive costs of fatal, hospitalized, and non-hospitalized traumatic brain injuries among civilians in 2000 alone was estimated to total more than $76.5 billion. This included $14.6 billion in medical costs and a significantly higher cost in work-related losses. An additional $137 billion was attributed to loss in quality of life.

In light of these statistics, it is apparent that continued research, advocacy, and exploration of further rehabilitative options are a necessity. Fortunately, in recent years, there has been as increased awareness of the impact of brain injuries due to exposure in things such as national sports leagues and returning military veterans.

10

Chapter 2
Tour of the Brain – Function and Injury

In this chapter we will explore the various regions of the brain, the roles they play, and the wide range of health concerns and symptoms that can arise from an injury to a certain brain area.

The Brain Stem and Cranial Nerves
Functional Overview
The brain stem is the most ancient of brain structures and lies at the root of our ability to survive and maintain life. It lies deep within the brain and can be divided into the following substructures:
-medulla oblongata (myencephalon)
-pons (metencephalon)
-midbrain (mesencephalon)
-reticular formation
-cranial nerves

Together the brain stem mediates and controls arousal, attention, heart rate, breathing, the sleep cycle, balance, gross movements, coordination of eye, jaw, tongue, and head movements. It also processes visual, sensory, digestive, and auditory perception. These functions operate in an automatic, rhythmic fashion without ever being thought about, needing neither conscious effort or the participation of higher brain structures. Basic motor movements such as sucking, chewing, swallowing, swimming, stepping and walking are also controlled by the brainstem.

Structures of the Brainstem		
Medulla		breathing, heart rate, blood pressure, automatic actions such as coughing, sneezing, swallowing, or vomiting
Pons		sleep, breathing, swallowing, bladder control, hearing, equilibrium, taste, eye movement, facial expressions, facial sensation, and posture, suspected role in dreaming and sleep paralysis.
Midbrain	Periaqueductal gray	motor-vocal aspects of emotional expression, laughing, crying, howling, plosive sounds, facial expressions
	Superior colliculi	multi-modal assimilation area orienting individual toward external stimuli and movement
	Inferior colliculus	detects and analyzes and localizes auditory stimuli of various sound sources
Reticular Formation		Integration of sensory input is received from the skin, muscles, joints, and vestibular system and coordination of responsive behavior

Medulla:
The medulla is the portion of the brainstem farthest back within the skull. Here are found what are known as spinal or pyramidal tracts which cross over between the brain and body to exchange information from the body to the opposite hemisphere of the brain. This is why the left side of the brain controls the right side of the body and vice versa.
Functions: automatic actions including breathing, heart rate, and blood pressure.
Reflex centers control automatic actions such as coughing, sneezing, swallowing, or vomiting.
If injured: Possible coma with accompanying heart and breathing disturbances
Associated cranial nerves: IX (glossiopharyngeal), X (vagus), XI (accessory), and XII (hypoglossal).

Pons:
The pons relays signals from the from brainstem to the cerebellum
Functions: sleep, breathing, swallowing, bladder control, hearing, equilibrium, taste, eye movement, facial expressions, facial sensation, and posture. It is thought to also play a role in dreaming, sleepwalking, and sleep paralysis.
Associated cranial nerves: V (trigeminal), VI (abducens), VII (facial), and VIII (vestibulocochlear).

Midbrain
The midbrain is the smallest part of the brainstem and can divided into three portions:
Tegmentum: outgrowth of the reticular formation and includes dopamine production neurons
The tectum: includes the superior (visual) and inferior (auditory) colliculi
Substania nigra: a major production source of dopamine. The "red nucleus" allows for flexor muscle tone.

The *periaqueductal gray* is also in the midbrain and receives extensive input from the limbic system/amygdala.
Functions: motor-vocal aspects of emotional expression, responses to painful or noxious stimuli, coordination of the laryngeal, oral-facial, and both primary and accessory muscles of breathing. These pre-programmed motor-vocal operations can produce a wide range of noises that generally sound like a negative mood, as well as plosive sounds such as "puh" "guh" "kuh"", etc. which require a strong puff also be made. These don't have anything do do with actual felt emotions. As long as the brainstem is active, someone can still laugh, cry, or howl; even if the rest of the brain is inactive. Injuries to areas controlling facial expression can cause loss of control of the face may contort in a manner of extreme happiness or grief despite not feeling these emotions.

Reticular Activating System
Functions: arousal and activation of the neuroaxis. Integrates sensory input received from the skin, muscles, joints, and vestibular system. This may be movements of the trunk, limbs, head, or eyes. Sensory-motor integration is mediated by the excitatory neurotransmitter glutamate, and the inhibitory neurotransmitter gamma-aminobutyric acid (GABA). Modulatory functions are mediated by norepinephrine and serotonin. If there is severe injury, a permanent comatose state can result.

Cranial Nerves

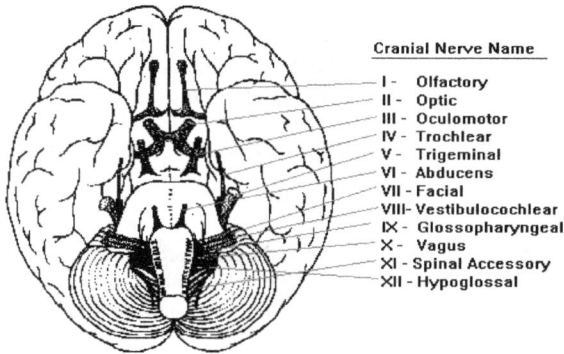

Cranial Nerve Name

I - Olfactory
II - Optic
III - Oculomotor
IV - Trochlear
V - Trigeminal
VI - Abducens
VII - Facial
VIII - Vestibulocochlear
IX - Glossopharyngeal
X - Vagus
XI - Spinal Accessory
XII - Hypoglossal

The Cranial Nerves – Pathology and Symptoms

I - Olfactory	Loss of smell/taste, risk of cerebrospinal fluid fistula
II - Optic	Visual defects including blindness, neglect, etc.
III - Oculomotor	Drooping eyelid, pupil unresponsive to direct light, inability to move eye downward, upward, or inward
IV - Trochlear	Inability to move eye in order to look in downward or inward direction
V - Trigeminal	Face pain, difficulty chewing, atrophy or paralysis of temporal or jaw muscles
VI - Abducens	Lateral gaze paralysis, horizontal diplopia
VII -Facial	Bells' Palsy, facial paralysis or flaccidity, eyebrow raising, eyelid closure paralysis, taste loss in anterior 2/3 of tongue, sounds may seem too loud or painful
VIII -Vestibular	Vertigo, nauea, dizziness, leaning or veering to one side when walking, unsteadiness, abnormal sensations of movement, tinnitus, nystagmus, difficulty focusing on objects when they are moving or when walking
IX -Glossopharyngeal	Loss of taste/sensation in posterior 1/3 of tongue, loss of gag reflex and carotid sinus reflex, painful swallowing or cough
X - Vagus	Pseudobulbar palsy, difficulty swallowing/dysphagia, slurred speech, palate weakness, gastroparesis, hyperarousal, smooth muscle cramping, IBS, weight gain, depression, bradycardia, chronic inflammation, nutritional deficiencies, seizures
XI – Spinal Accessory	Ipsilateral sagging shoulder(s), weakness in turning head (esp. against resistance)
XII - Hypoglossal	Tongue weakness/atropy/deviation

I – Olfactory Nerve

Not a cranial nerve, in the strictest sense, as it bypasses the brainstem, the olfactory nerve projects to many other brain structures. It is, however, associated with many brainstem functions as it receives information about smell and taste. If an injury occurs the nerve may become severed, and the meninges may rupture. If this happens someone may lose their sense of smell (asnosmia) and possibly also develop a cerebrospinal fistula in which cerebrospinal fluid drips or gushes into the nose. Dysosmia, or a problem in sense of smell may also occur due to partial injuries.

II - Optic Nerve

Visual signals from the retina of the eye to the brain are transmitted via the optic nerves. Injuries to these pathways result in visual defects. Defects to both eyes suggest either an injury to both hemispheres of the brain or to the retina or optic nerve before entering the skull. Complete destruction of the optic tract results in visual neglect to the left or right, whereas a partial injury may create a quadratic visual defect in which a quadrant of the visual field is affected.

III – Oculomotor Nerve

Innervation of all rotary muscles of the eye, with the exception of two, is provided by the oculomotor nerve. This includes the muscles along the top, bottom, and area near the bridge of the nose. Also controlled are the muscles of the pupil (ciliary and pupilloconstrictor muscles), and the muscle that raises the eyelid (levator palprebrae). If damaged there may be an inability to rotate the eye upward, downward, or inward. The pupil may also not respond to direct light and there may be drooping of the eyelid (ptosis).

IV – Trochlear Nerve

Innervates the superior oblique muscle of the eye letting someone look downward and inward by controlling depression, abduction and intorsion of the eyeball. This is the most common cranial nerve to be damaged from head trauma.

V – Trigeminal

The largest of the cranial nerves, it control the ability to close the jaw, chew, and movement of the jaw from side to side. Along with the facial nerve, it controls facial expression. Injury to this nerve can cause difficulty in chewing. In severe cases muscle weakening of one side and complete paralysis of the muscles of the side of the jaw can occur. Portions of the nerve take in sensory input such as temperature, touch, and pain from the face, teeth, mouth, and mucus membranes of the nose, cheek, tongue and sinuses. The sometimes intensely painful condition known as trigeminal neuralgia is an instance of this.

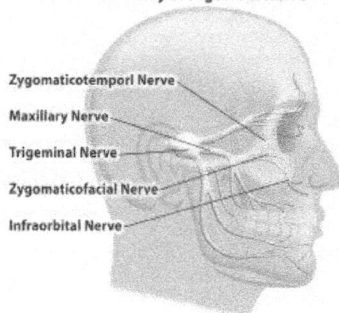

Anatomy of Trigeminal Nerve

Zygomaticotempori Nerve
Maxillary Nerve
Trigeminal Nerve
Zygomaticofacial Nerve
Infraorbital Nerve

VI -Abducens

Mostly concerned with horizontal eye movement. An injury can cause lateral gaze paralysis or paralysis of the lateral rectus muscle which results in horizontal double vision (diplopia).

14

VII – Facial
In charge of movement of the face. This includes the ability to raise eyebrows, movement of the lips, closure of the auditory canals and digestive sensation. The facial nerve also innervates the taste buds of the front 2/3 of the tongue, which if injured, can cause a loss of taste. Also innervated is the stapedius muscle, which helps dampen noise. If the stapedius becomes paralyzed, an individual may experience sounds as too loud, intolerable or painful. Other symptoms associated with an injury to this nerve include lip retraction, eyebrow lifting, eyelid closure paralysis (Bell's Palsy), inability to wrinkle one's forehead, purse their lips or show their teeth or there be drooping of the corner of the mouth.

VIII – Vestibular
The vestibular portion of the 8th cranial nerve innervates the inner ear. The primary function of this nerve is to determine the body's position in space to maintain balance during movement. If there is an injury to the vestibular receptors, there can be abnormal sensations of movement, vertigo, nausea, tendencies to fall, dizziness, and motion sickness. Hearing problems including deafness or hearing a buzzing, humming, whistling, roaring, hissing or clicking sound (tinnitus) can also occur. They may feel as though they are being pulled to one side or lean/veer to one side when walking. Difficulty focusing one's vision when moving or when an object is in motion (nystagmus) can occur as well.

IX – Glossopharyngeal
Closely related to the vagus nerve, the 9th cranial nerve receives tactile, thermal, and pain sensations from the tongue. It also receives information about carotid artery pressure. All of this information is transmitted to the vagus nerve. Together, the 9th and 10th cranial nerves can influence heart rate and arterial blood pressure. Injuries will usually result in loss of taste and sensation in the back 1/3 of the tongue, a loss of gag reflex, and carotid sinus reflex. Swallowing or coughing may become intensely painful.

X – Vagus
Actually a complex mix of nerves, the vagus innervates a number of structures including the throat (larynx, pharynx, trachea, epiglottis), esophagus, and internal organs. As such, important bodily functions such as swallowing, breathing, speaking, and movement of the palate are all within its influence. An injury can cause palate weakness and pseudobulbal palsy. Speech can be severely affected as well, becoming excessively nasally if fluids get into the nasal passages. Due to it's long-reaching influence on a wide range of structures many other symptoms may develop from injury, including paralysis of the digestive tract (gastroparesis), hyperarousal, smooth muscle cramping, IBS, weight gain, depression, bradycardia, chronic inflammation, nutritional deficiencies, and seizures.

XI – Spinal Accessory Nerve
There are two distinct segments of this nerve. The cranial portion helps control the larynx. The spinal portion of this nerve innervates the sternocleidomastoid (SCM) and upper trapezius muscles to help turn the head and elevate the shoulders. An injury to this nerve may cause one's shoulders to sag on the affected side or weakness in turning the head.

XII – Hypoglossal Nerve
This nerve controls movement of the tongue. If the nerve is damaged, the muscles of the tongue will weaken and atrophy. Tongue strength can be tested by placing one's tongue on one side of the cheek and pressing against a finger placed on the outside of the cheek.

Brainstem: Activities for activation

-Smell and taste food
-Speech, phonation, "ah", singing
-Facial movements
-Corneal puffs
-Palate stimulation/gum rolls in mouth
-Jaw exercises

The Cerebellum

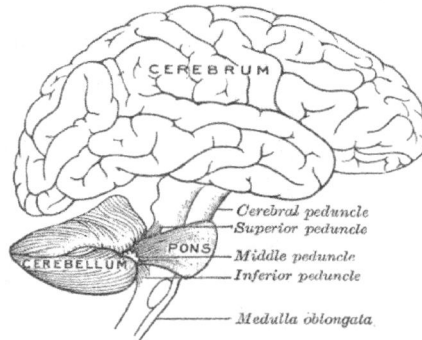

Cerebral peduncle
Superior peduncle
Middle peduncle
Inferior peduncle
Medulla oblongata

Functional Overview

The cerebellum sits atop the brainstem. It accounts for approximately 25% of overall brain volume. While most commonly associated with motor movements and their smoothness of action, the cerebellum has also been shown to be involved in cognitive, emotional, sensory, and speech processing. It communicates with almost all other regions of the brain, with the exception of the striatum. Neuroplasticity has been demonstrated here, as have functions of learning and memory. It has been theorized that the cerebellum may serve as an integrative interface for cognition, emotion, motor functioning and memory.

The Cerebellum – Pathology and Symptoms

Motor Movement	-Gait ataxia -Vertigo -Hypotonia -Intention tremor -Abnormalties in force, accuracy, range, and rate of goal directed movements -Lack of motor coordination (asynergia) -Inability to make fast alternating movements of the limbs (dysdiachokinesia) -Involuntary motor sequences
Visual and verbal	-Disrupted visually tracking of movements and determination of movement trajectory: past pointing; distances are incorrectly judged -Falling short or going too far trying to touch/grasp an object (dysmetria) -Involuntary slow and fast rhythmic lateral eye movements usually to the side of the lesion (nystagmus) -Dysarthric speech -Difficulty with paired verbal testing
Emotional	-Increased "rage response" (semi-purposeful/"sham") -Hyperactivity -Autonomic function dysregulation (heart rate, blood pressure, breathing, gastromotility, etc) -Possible schizophrenia psychoses -Possible autistic-like symptoms

Motor Functions
As far as motor control, the cerebellum helps coordinate, smooth, fine tune, and maintain timing of motor movements. Activity in some deeper structures can fire by just thinking about making a movement.

Dystaxia, predominantly in the legs, can result from cerebellar dysfunction. This can often appear to others as if the individual is heavily intoxicated. In fact, in addition to trauma, drinking alcohol and nutritional deficiencies can result in damage to the cerebellum. Motor related disturbances including tremor, nystagmus, gait disturbances, lack of coordination, and postural instability can be common following an injury.

When you acquire a new skilled movement, such as playing a guitar or a piano, it requires conscious control of your movements and much more activity of the neocortex while the cerebellum plays a minimal role. With practice, less conscious attention is needed, and "motor memory" becomes more prominent. Over time, the cerebellum begins to take control over the task, operating subconsciously, with little or no help from the forebrain. Lesions can make this ability difficult or not possible. Compound movements are more severely affected than simple movements.

The lateral cerebellum involves regulating the timing of sequential movements. An injury causes difficulty with maintaining timing and rhythm. Abnormalities in the rate, range, and force of movement are seen as deficiencies in finger to nose testing. Irregularities in speeding up and slowing down movement are also common. When asked to make movements as fast as possible someone will often do so slower than normal.

Cerebellar Gait
What is referred to as "cerebellar gait" is typically seen with a wide based gait, steps being characteristically unsteady, irregular, uncertain, and of variable length. If mild it may only be noticeable when tired, if severe it may not be possible to stand without assistance.
Symptoms may include:
-Loss of muscle tone
-Lack of coordination in volitional movements
-Intention tremor
-Minor degrees of muscle weakness
-Easily fatigued
-Disorders of equilibrium including nystagmus are common features.

Language Functions
The newer parts of the cerebellum contribute to and are concerned with cognitive functioning including language. The right cerebellum (interconnected with the left cerebral hemisphere) becomes activated when asked to produce verbs in response to nouns. The cerebellum also becomes activated when reading aloud as opposed to looking at words. Moving the mouth without speaking also activates the cerebellum, whereas internal (silent) speech without motor movement does not.

Those with cerebellar injuries may have trouble with verbal paired association tests. With severe injuries there may be initial mutism.

Ataxic Speech
Speech can also be affected and become "dysarthric". This may be of two types:

-Slowed and slurred, particularly when required to repeat sounds ("ga ga ga")
-Scanning dysarthria as words are broken up into syllables, some of which are explosively uttered (i.e. "ballistic speech").

Vision and Visuo-spatial Functions
Motor tasks may become troublesome when visual cues generally used to guide movement are eliminated.

Emotional Activity
Injury and electrical stimulation of the cerebellum have shown emotional responses including strong emotions like rage and constant states of hyperactivity. Stimulation of the front portion of the cerebellum will elicit rage-like reactions including threat, attack, and autonomic changes such as blood pressure/heart rate changes, goosebumps, dilation of the pupils, urination, or gastrointestinal changes. These do not tend to be directed at anything in particular and thus may be referred to as "sham rage." The back portion of the cerebellum has the exact opposite effect.

These emotional responses of the cerebellum tend to mostly be due to rich interconnections with the limbic system (explored later in this chapter). It is hypothesized that the cerebellum might inhibit the limbic system. Emotional and affective behavior with autonomic changes also appear to be influenced by connections with the brainstem. Abnormalities in the cerebellum have also been implicated in the origin of cases of schizophrenia and autism; as well as post-injury/surgery mutism and highly abnormal emotional behavior that will often resolve after a few days or weeks. It has been noted that up to 50% of patients diagnosed as psychotic or schizophrenic conditions display cerebellar abnormalities, including atrophy of the vermis or tumors and approximately 50% of those who are psychotically depressed show a similar pattern of cerebellar abnormality.

Cerebellum: Activities for activation

General Cerebellum
-Warming auditory canal (same side)
-Revolving chair movement (side of direction)
-Passive muscle stretch (same side)
-Squeezing tennis ball (same side)
-Eye movement up the affected side and down unaffected side
-Pointing with hand of affected side

Medial Cerebellum
-Gym ball exercises, wobble board, balance mat
-Gyroscope
-Bouncing ball against ground
-Visual fixation with head rotation

Lateral Cerebellum
-Questions leading to a "yes" answer
-Learning a musical instrument
-Tracing a maze
-Throwing and catching a ball against a wall
-Tapping to beat of music/metronome
 -Voluntary motor movement
-Trying to write with eyes closed
-Board games involving strategy/planning
-Silently generating verbs and reading nouns aloud

The Occipital Lobe

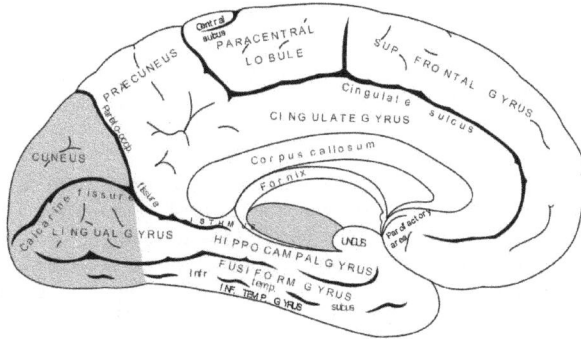

Functional Overview

The occipital lobe is composed of two basic subsections: the primary visual cortex and the visual association area. Simple and complex visual analysis is one of the main functions of the occipital lobe, however neurons also tend to a number of other functions including vestibular, sound, sight, visceral, and sensory input. These are subdivided into 4 visual cortices:

The primary visual cortex (V1)
V1 is concerned with the elementary aspects of form perception, transforming information from the retina into a basic code that enables visual information to be extracted by later processing. It is particularly specialized in processing spatial information such as static and moving stimuli, colors, and pattern recognition. This is the most ancient visual portion of the brain and found in most mammals.

Prestriate cortex (V2)
Receiving strong connections from V1, V2 neurons are similar and are tuned to simple properties such as orientation, spatial frequency, size and color. In addition to further processing these qualities, V2 neurons also process more complex properties like orientation of illusionary contours, discrepancies between information coming from the two eyes, whether objects are part of the foreground or background, and some attention maintenance. The deepest layer of this area has been found to play an important role in the storage of object recognition memory and the conversion of short-term object memories into long term memories.

Third visual complex (V3)
Located immediately in front of V2, some subdivide this area even further into dorsal and ventral portions, V3A, and V3B respectively. The dorsal V3 region receives input from V1 and V2 and may play a role in global or coherent motion of large patterns. The ventral V3 region has weaker connections from V1 and is more connected with the inferior temporal lobe.

Fourth visual area (V4)
Receives strong input from V2 and some input from V1 and seems to be the first brain region to show strong attentional modulation and selective attention. Similar to V1, V4

responds to orientation, spatial frequency and color; however it also processes more complex features such as geometric shapes. V4 is believed to be the main color center in the brain due to lesions resulting in lack of color vision.

Visual area 5 (V5), aka middle temporal visual area (MT)
V5 is specialized in assessing the movement of objects. 90% of cells in this region respond to only a single direction of movement and will not respond if movement is in the opposite direction. Damage to this area of the brain can cause an inability to gauge movement or speed. Perception may feel like a series of pictures rather than a fluid experience.

Once visual information has been processed by the occipital lobe, it is next relayed to the parietal lobe and to the inferior temporal lobe, where higher order analysis and processing can happen. Damage to the parietal-occipital borders can result in troubles with form and depth perception, as well as visual neglect. Injury to the temporal-occipital regions can give rise to visual agnosias and an inability to recognize complex objects and faces.

The occipital lobes also appear to be lateralized in certain functions such as facial recognition. For example, destruction of the right occipital region is associated with face blindness (prosopagnosia), and abnormal activity in this area is more likely to give rise to complex visual hallucinations.

Pathology & Symptoms

Cortical Blindness
Prosopagnosia (Face Blindness)
Occipital lesions, especially of the entire visual cortex

Symptoms:
Inability to discriminate between changes between light and darkness

If restricted to only one hemisphere: loss of patterned vision for the opposite half of the visual field (hemianopsia).
If only part of the visual cortex is damaged: vision loss is only in the corresponding quadrant of the visual field (scatoma). In cases of partial cortical blindness, someone is usually able to make compensatory eye movements and are not terribly troubled by the disability. Often someone may not even be aware of loss of a quadrant or even half of their visual field. Because of this, it should be tested for.

Differential Diagnosis

Right temporal-occipital region:
-Disturbance in the ability to recognize the faces of self, friends, loved ones, or pets
-Inability to discriminate and identify even facial affect

Inferior and middle temporal lobe:
-Loss of the ability to recognize faces
-Disturbances in visual discrimination learning and retention
-Visual closure difficulty & recognizing different shapes and patterns or objects which differ in regard to size or color

Posterior right temporal region:
-Disrupts visual-spatial memory for faces in general
-Inability to correctly label emotion faces

Visual Agnosia "Blind Sight"

Visual preservation after an injury to V1 has been referred to as "blind sight".
Although blind, theys may avoid obstacles, retrieve desired objects, and can thus appear to have some residual visual function despite claiming to not have any sense of sight.
This may be due to unaffected processing areas of V5 involved in visual orientation. With occipital lesions, complex visual input may still reach the temporal lobe and be directed onward to the auditory areas through a secondary route so that "feelings" of seeing something can be communicated and objects can be named, but the person denies visual perception.

Apperceptive visual agnosia:
A disturbance in perceptual and visual-motor integration (difficulty copying or matching objects, failing to draw the complete object). Someone is able to trace but not able to recognize where they started. Inability to place visual details into an integral whole, recognizing only isolated details. If unnecessary lines are drawn across the picture, the ability to recognize the object deteriorates further.
Associated with parietal occipital cortex or bilateral damage to the inferior-occipital cortex

Associative visual agnosia:
A deficit in naming in which sounds cannot be matched to a visual perception. May also have inability to read (alexa)
Associated with left inferior/middle temporal, parietal occipital cortex, or occipital injuries.

Simultanagnosia:
An inability to see more than one thing, or all aspects of an item, at a time.
Associated with bilateral superior occipital lobe or superior occipital-parietal injuries

Impaired Color Recognition Denial Of Blindness

While sometimes able to correctly name objects, an individual cannot correctly name, match, and identify or point to colors. Prosopanosia is also frequently displayed.

-23% of those with right cerebral damage and 12% of those with left sided destruction had trouble with color matching.
-Impairments of color perception are often secondary to bilateral inferior occiptial lobe damage.
-Almost 50% of those with aphasia demonstrate deficient color naming and color identification.

People with cortical blindness seem initially confused, indifferent about their condition, and report a variety of hallucinatory experiences that can range from simple to complex. Often they will initially deny that they experience any blindness and confabulate (Anton's syndrome). It is possible they deny being blind because subcortically they are still able to see and be aware of the visual world, but at a neocortical level there is no sight.

Visual Hallucinations
When portions of the temporal lobe or occipital lobe are damaged, disconnected, or compromised, the ability to store information or draw visual-verbal imagery from memory is severely impacted. When artificially or abnormally activated, visual-auditory imagery and a variety of other involuntary emotions can happen. These may include complex hallucinations, dream-like states, episodes of confusion, or placing emotional significance to otherwise neutral thoughts and external experiences.

Hallucinations may occur secondarily to tumors or seizures involving the occipital, parietal, frontal, and temporal lobe. They can also arise after toxic exposure, high fevers, general infections, exhaustion, starvation, extreme thirst, and with partial or complete blindness such as due to glaucoma. Individuals suffering from cortical blindness frequently experience hallucinations.

Hallucinations secondary to loss of visual or auditory input seems to be the brain's interpretation of neural noise. When there is lack of input, various areas of the brain begin to extract or assign significance to random neural events, or to whatever limited input may be coming in. Conversely, hallucinations can also happen due to increased levels of neural noise.

With anterior and inferior temporal abnormalities, the hallucinations become increasing complex, consisting of both auditory and visual features, including faces, people, objects, animals, etc. This gives rise to the most complex forms of imagery. Even more, structures such as the amygdala and hippocampus become activated and can result in evoking memories and emotions. So much so that the experience may become personally meaningful to include real individuals and real events that are produced from memory.

Differential Diagnosis of Visual Hallucinations

Middle Temporal Lobe
Tumors or electrical stimulation: associated with the development of auditory and visual hallucinations, dreamy states, and alterations in emotional functioning

Occipital Lobe
Striate Cortex (V1, Brodmann's area 17)
simple visual hallucinations such as:
-Sparks
-Tongues of flames
-Colors and flashes of lights
-Objects may seem to become exceedingly large (macropsia) or small (micropsia)
-Blurred outlines
-Stretched out in a single dimension
-Colors may become modified or even erased
-Sometimes simple geometric forms

Visual Association Areas (brodmann's Areas 18 & 19)
complex visual hallucinations such as:

-Images of men or animals
-Various objects and geometric figures
-Individuals with smaller or larger than usual features
-Objects may seem to become telescoped/far away, or, when approached, objects may seem to loom and become exceedingly large.

Complex hallucinations are usually quite vivid and fully formed to where they may be thought of as real. Although usually associated with tumors or abnormal activation of the visual association area, complex hallucinations have also been reported with parietal-occipital involvement, occipital-temporal, or inferior-temporal damage, or with injury to the occipital pole and convexity.
Laterality: complex hallucinations are usually associated with right rather than left-sided injuries.

Occipital Lobe: Activities for activation

-Spatial orientation
-Vertical movements in the same side visual field

The Limbic System

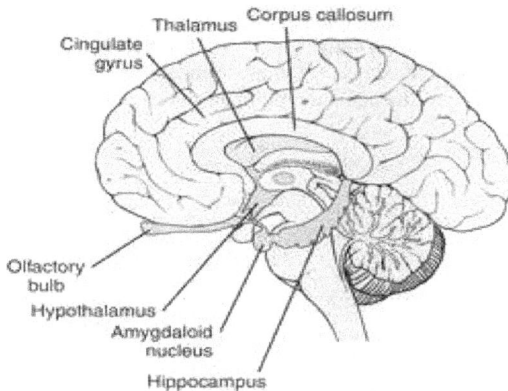

Labels on diagram: Cingulate gyrus, Thalamus, Corpus callosum, Olfactory bulb, Hypothalamus, Amygdaloid nucleus, Hippocampus

Functional Overview

Buried within the cerebrum lie several large structures that make up the limbic system. These are preeminent in the control and mediation of memory, emotion, learning, dreaming, attention, arousal, and the perception and expression of emotional, motivational, sexual, and social behavior. This includes the formation of loving attachments. The limbic brain has become less prominent as the forebrain has evolutionarily grown in use. It has not been replaced however, as it is not only predominant in regard to all aspects of motivational and emotional functioning, but is capable of completely overtaking the "rational mind". This is due in part to the massive axonal projections of the limbic system into the neocortex.

The major structures of the limbic system include the hypothalamus, amygdala, hippocampus, septal nuclei, and anterior cingulate gyrus; structures which are directly interconnected by massive axonal pathways.

Hypothalamus

This could be considered the most "primitive" aspect of the limbic system, despite being exceedingly complex. A primary function of the hypothalamus is the regulation of the autonomic nervous system which controls most automatic, unconscious functions within the body. The hypothalamus integrates autonomic responses and endocrine function with behavior to maintain homeostasis of certain systems. Blood pressure and electrolyte balance are maintained by thirst and salt appetite. Body temperature is regulated by control of metabolic changes and heat or cool seeking behaviors. Energy metabolism is regulated by eating, digestion, and metabolic rate. Reproduction is regulated through hormonal control. Emergency responses to stress are controlled by regulating blood flow to muscles and the release of adrenal stress hormones. The medial hypothalamus controls parasympathetic activities (e.g. reduction in heart rate, increased peripheral circulation) and has a dampening effect on certain forms of emotional/motivational arousal. The lateral hypothalamus mediates sympathetic activity (increasing heart rate, elevation of blood pressure) and is involved in controlling the metabolic and bodily responses of heightened emotionality.

Nearly every region of the cerebrum interacts with and can be influenced by the hypothalamus. The hypothalamus uses its blood supply to carry hormonal messages to the bodily organs and other brain structures. The blood supply and cerebrospinal fluid are used to receive information as well, bypassing the synaptic route nearly all other regions of the neuroaxis use. It is exceedingly responsive to the sense of smell. The information received is sensory information from all over the body, which is then compared with biologic set points. If an abnormality is found, it adjusts autonomic, endocrine, and behavioral responses to return to a healthy balance by influencing the pituitary gland and hormonal secretion.

Regions of the Hypothalamus			
Region	Area	Nucleus	Function
Anterior	Medial	Medial preoptic nucleus	Regulates the release of gonadotropic hormones from the adenohypophysis. Contains the sexually dimorphic nucleus, which releases GnRH.
		Supraoptic nucleus •	Oxytocin release, Vasopressin release
		Paraventricular nucleus•	Corticotropin-releasing hormone
		Anterior hypothalamic • nucleus	Thermoregulation, panting, sweating, thyrotropin inhibition
		Suprachiasmic nucleus •	Vasopressin release, circadian rhythms
	Lateral	Lateral preoptic nucleus	
		Lateral Nucleus •	Thirst and hunger
		Part of supraoptic nucleus	Vasopressin release
Tuberal	Medial	Dorsomedial hypothalamic nucleus	Blood pressure, heart rate, GI stimulation
		Ventromedial nucleus	Satiety, neuroendocrine control
		Arcuate nucleus	Growth hormone releleasing hormone (GHRH), feeding, dopamine
	Lateral	Lateral nucleus	Thirst, hunger
		Lateral tuberal nuclei	
Posterior	Medial	Mammillary nuclei	Memory
		Posterior nucleus	Increased blood pressure, pupillary dilation, shivering
	Lateral	Lateral nucleus	

Hormone	Effect
Thyrotropin-releasing hormone (TRH)	-Stimulates thyroid-stimulating hormone (TSH) release from anterior pituitary -Stimulate prolactin release from anterior pituitary
Dopamine (DA)	-Inhibits prolactin release from anterior pituitary
Growth hormone-releasing hormone (GRHR)	Stimulates Growth hormone (GH) release from anterior pituitary
Somatostatin (SS)	Inhibits Growth hormone (GH) release from anterior pituitary Inhibits thyroid-stimulating hormone (TSH) release from anterior pituitary
Gonadotrophin – releasing hormone (GnRH)	-Stimulates follicle-stimulating hormone (FSH) release from anterior pituitary -Stimulate luteinizing hormone (LH) release from anterior pituitary

Corticotropin-releasing hormone (CRH)	-Stimulates adrenocorticotropic hormone (ACTH) release from anterior pituitary
Oxytocin	-Uterine contraction -Lactation (letdown reflex)
Vasopressin/antidiuretic hormone (ADH)	Increase in the permeability to water of the cells of distal tubuleand collecting duct in the kidney, allowing water reabsorption and excretion of concentrated urine

	Possible Symptoms Associated with Lateral vs Medial Hypothalamic Damage
Lateral Lesion	-No motivation to eat or drink (Aphagia, adipsia) -Lessened sense of pleasure and emotional responsiveness -Pathological laughter and crying -Passiveness, inability to become aggressive
Medial Lesion	-Excessive eating, severe obesity (especially ventromedial) -Pathological laughter and crying -Aggressive or attack behavior, rage-like outbursts, propensity toward violence

Amygdala

The amygdala has been associated with generating both the most basic and most profound of human emotions including fear, sexual desire, rage, and religious ecstasy. At a more basic level, it aids in determining if something might be appropriate to eat. The amygdala is involved in the seeking out of loving attachments and the formation of long term emotional memories. It contains neurons which become activated by the human face and in response to the direction of someone else's gaze. Chemical systems in the amygdala include opiate, leutenizing hormone, vasopressin, somatostatin, and corticotropin releasing factor. The amygdala can be likened to the chief executive of the limbic system, wielding enormous power over the impulses of the hypothalamus. The amygdala is also directly connected to the hippocampus, with which it interacts to play a role in memory storage. It particularly plays a role in the emotional significance of memories. The influence of the amygdala can become so substantial that it is able to overwhelm the neocortex and assume control over behavior when emotions run high.

The amygdala is buried within the depths of the anterior-inferior temporal lobe and consists of several major groups. The medial group (cortico-medial amygdala) is involved in smell, sexuality, and motor activity. In females, the medial amygdala is a principle site for uptake of the female sex hormone, estrogen, and contains a high concentration of leutenizing hormone which plays an important role during pregnancy and nursing. This region is also rich in cells containing endorphins (enkephalins), and opiate receptors can be found throughout the amygdala. This results in the amygdala becoming exceedingly active when experiencing a craving for pleasurable experiences and addictive drives such as sex, gambling, and/or drugs.

The lateral portion of the amygdala is the most cortex-like, relying on excitatory neurotransmitters, such as glutamate. This is intimately involved in all aspects of emotional activity and is very important in analyzing information and transferring it back to the neocortex for further processing. The lateral division controls the emotional meaning and significance being assigned to, as well as extracted from, that which is experienced.

27

Possible Symptoms Associated with Amygdala Injury
-Docility (hypoactivity) -Intractible aggression or fear (hyperactivity) -Inability to recognize faces -Blunted emotions -Lack of emotional speech -Inability to appropriately respond to social-emotional stimuli (social-emotional agnosia) -Difficulty maintaining attention -Inability to sing, convey melodic information or to properly enunciate via vocal inflection (right sided injury) -Prolonged, repeated, and inappropriate sexual behavior and/or masturbation -High risk behavior, reduced loss aversion (e.g. gambling) -Memory deficits -Tendency to react to every stimuli -Tendency to put objects into the mouth

Hippocampus ("Ammon's Horn" or the "sea horse")
Functions of the hippocampus include components of memory, new learning, mental mapping of the environment, voluntary movement toward a goal, attention, behavioral arousal, and orienting reactions. It plays an exceedingly important role in memory, acting to place various short-term memories into long-term storage. Presumably the hippocampus encodes new information during the storage and consolidation (long-term storage) phase, and assists in the gating of information headed to the frontal lobe by filtering or suppressing irrelevant sense data that could interfere with memory consolidation. When information is repeatedly experienced, the hippocampus habituates. Thus, as information is attended to, recognized, and presumably learned and/or stored in memory, the role of the hippocampus becomes less.

The left amygdala and hippocampus are highly involved in processing and/or attending to verbal information, whereas the right amygdala/hippocampus is more involved in the learning, memory and recollection of non-verbal, visual-spatial, environmental, emotional, motivational, tactile, olfactory, and facial information. There is a minimal hippocampal involvement in emotions, though electrical stimulation has caused sensations of "anxiety" or "bewilderment". There is evidence that the hippocampus may also work to reduce extremes in stress hormone arousal.

Possible Symptoms Associated with Hippocampal Injury
-Impaired memory – inability to convert short term memories into long term memories (anterograde amnesia) -Impaired memory for words, passages, conversations, and written material (especially with left side injury) -Distractability -Hyperresponsiveness – may feel overwhelmed or confused as a result -Impairment in attention and learning -Disinhibition of behavioral responsiveness or shifting of attention -"Input overload" - the neuroaxis is overwhelmed by neural noise, disrupting memory consolidation to where information is not stored or even attended to

Septal Nuclei
The septal nuclei is, in part, an evolutionary and developmental outgrowth of the hippocampus and the hypothalamus. It links these two structures along with the amygdala, brainstem, and the sustania innomminata, which is a major memory center, that manufactures Acetylcholine (ACh) -a transmitter directly implicated in memory. These interconnections are thought to allow the septal nuclei to modulate memory functioning and arousal in the hippocampus. The septal nuclei is also connected with and shares a counterbalancing relationship with the amygdala, particularly regarding emotional and sexual arousal. For example, where the amygdala promotes indiscriminate contact seeking, and perhaps promiscuous sexual activity, the septal nuclei inhibits these tendencies, helping in the formation of selective and more enduring emotional attachments. The septal nuclei can also produce extremes of emotion, including explosive violence, known as "septal rage."

Possible Symptoms Associated with Septal Nuclei Injury
-Memory loss (acetylcholine, norepinephrine, and serotonin loss in the hippocampus) -Difficulty remembering one's surroundings -Difficulty with learning and memory due to abolishment of hippocampal theta states -Increased emotionality or aggression -"Septal rage" - hyper-emotionality, rage, hyperactivity, increased eating

Anterior Cingulate
The anterior cingulate is considered a transitional cortex. It is intimately interconnected with the hypothalamus, amygdala, septal nuclei, and hippocampus, participating in memory and emotion including the experience of pain, misery, and anxiety. The evolution and expression of maternal behavior is also directly related to this structure. The anterior cingulate is the most vocal aspect of the brain, becoming active during language tasks, and generating emotional-melodic aspects of speech. These are because of connections with the bilateral frontal speech areas and the vocalization center in the midbrain (periaqueductal grey). Because of this, the anterior cingulate is involved in more cognitive aspects of social-emotional behavior including language and the establishment of long term attachments, beginning with the mother-infant bond. This structure is sexually differentiated which likely contributes to differences in melodic speech pattern differences between males and females. The possibilities of "maternal" vs. "paternal" behavior tendencies being rooted within these differentiations has been proposed.

Possible Symptoms Associated with Anterior Cingulate Injury
-Anxiety/panic disorder -Apathy/blunted emotions -Depressive symptoms -Lack of emotional speech -Social and emotional inappropriateness or unresponsiveness -Stuttering, word repetition, uncontrollably babbling or (if severe) mutism

Olfactory Bulb
The olfactory bulb and olfactory system are also implicated in the functioning of the limbic

system, the limbic striatum (nucleus accumbens, olfactory tubercle, substantia innominata, ventral caudate and putamen), the orbital frontal and inferior temporal lobes, along with the midbrain monoamine system. These systems and structures are also directly connected or separated by only a single synapse, which tend to become aroused not only as a function of emotional arousal, but in reaction to smell. In this way, the olfactory bulb and one's sense of smell continues to exert strong effects on the limbic system and on human behavior.

The Parietal Lobes

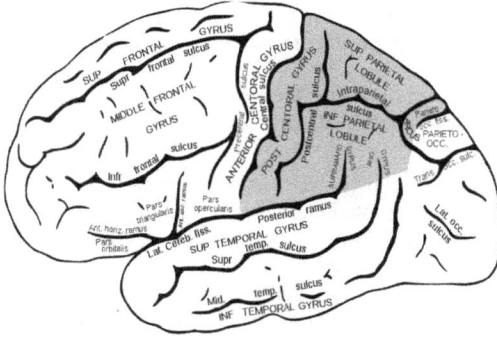

Functional Overview

The parietal lobes maintain an individuals body image and perception of the body. While commonly associated with the sense of touch and sensation, they are also concerned with motor and attentional functioning, the perception of spatial relations including depth, orientation, location, and identifying significant auditory, sensory, and visual stimuli. Distinct sensory signals are received from the entire body providing information about one's surroundings.

The parietal lobe guides the movement of the body in space, coordinating body movements while running, walking, climbing, etc through dense interconnections between primary somesthetic with the motor areas in the frontal lobe and signals sent down the spinal cord. The parietal lobes are also considered the primary structure relating to the hand as it receives sensations from the bones, tendons, muscles, and skin of the hand, then guiding the movement of the hand within visual-space. This allows for someone to be able to reach for and manipulate tools, open and remove bottle caps and pour the contents into a glass.

The left inferior parietal lobe appears to be the central area concerned with skilled time-sequencing motor acts. These assist in programming the motor frontal cortex where the actions are actually executed. If the inferior parietal region is destroyed, the individual loses the ability to perform actions in an appropriate sequence or to even realize they have performed an action incorrectly. This condition is referred to as apraxia.

In contrast, right parietal injuries are associated with severe disturbances of emotion, constructional deficiencies, and a host of visual-spatial abnormalities including left sided neglect. For instance, when drawing pictures they may fail to draw the left half of an object, when writing or reading they may ignore the left half of words or the left half of the page. They may fail to perceive and respond to individuals standing to their left, or even the left half of their own body.

Injuries to the parietal lobe seldom affect one particular quadrant, or even remain restricted to the parietal lobe. Damage may be parietal-occipital, parietal-temporal, frontal-parietal, or even bilateral. Therefore, symptoms may vary such as showing agraphia but normal reading, stereognosis in the absence of apraxia, or varied mixtures of seemingly unrelated symptoms.

31

Primary Somesthetic Receiving Areas (Brodmann's areas 3ab,1,2)
This region consists of three narrow strips of tissue (areas 3ab, 1, 2) which differ in sensory input, each maintaining a complete and independent representation of the body.

Area 3a: Receives input from opposite side muscles & signals muscle flexion or extension
Area 3b: Receives opposite side signals from the skin

These are semi-independent and organized based on the parts which are most frequently stimulated, creating more representation on the brain in accordance with their sensory importance as shown in figure 2. The area devoted to the fingers, in fact, is 100 times larger than the area devoted to the trunk. This information is then relayed to the adjacent areas 1, and 2. Together these four strips of tissue form a functional unit that is responsive to touch, texture, shape, motion, and the direction of movement, including time-sequential patterning, and can directly monitor the position and movement of the extremities.

Area 1: Maintains an overlapping skin-joint body map
Area 2: Maintains a map of the joints and can signal the position and posture of the limbs based on input from the muscles

The right parietal area is dominant in many aspects of processing sensory information. Neurons in this half of the brain appear to be more sensitive and more responsive with a greater ability to monitor events occurring on either half of the body, but particularly the left. Because of this the left half of the body tends to be more sensitive than the right.

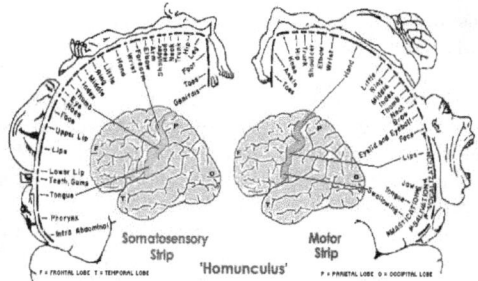

Somatosensory Strip   Motor Strip   'Homunculus'

Somesthetic (Supplementary) Association Area
This region controls and contains representations of both halves of the body. Bilateral representation is mostly maintained in the right half of the brain. A detailed representation of the skin surface, in particular the hand and face, is maintained here. A small percentage of cells also appear to be concerned with more complex activities such as the movement of the hand and arm and the manipulation of objects. Other neurons in this area are especially responsive in determining direction and rhythm of movement.

Polymodal Receiving Area (Area 7 and superior-posterior parietal)
This region is concerned with the analysis and integration of the highest order visual, auditory and sensory information. Through this it is able to create a three-dimensional image of the body in space. It guides gaze and whole body-positional movement, constantly updating information about internal and external coordinates. Neurons are thought to respond to signals transmitted from the limbic system (cingulate gyrus), middle and inferior temporal lobe. These cells guide and monitor eye movement so that the object of interest is fixated on, then motor movements, guiding the hand toward the object until it is grasped.

32

Connections with the parahippocampal gyrus allows for topographic learning in which cells can determine:

-Motivational significance
-Direction of movement
-Distance
-Spatial location
-Figure-ground relationships
-Depth: discrimination and determination of an objects 3-dimensional position in space

Posterior Parietal Areas 5, 7, & Supramarginal Gyrus
This region, in addition to sensory information, may also convey pain sensations. Neurons located in area 5 and 7 of the parietal lobe demonstrate pain sensitivity, with some area 7 neurons responding exclusively to thermal and painful stimuli with area 5 presumably acting to determine the source of pain.

Inferior parietal lobe / multimodal-assimilation area (Areas 7, 39, 40)
This part of the inferior parietal lobe has auditory and (in the left hemisphere) language capabilities. A single neuron simultaneously receives highly processed sensory, visual, auditory and movement related information from various association areas. They are involved in the capacity for the organization, labeling and multiple categorization of sensory-motor and conceptual events. This region becomes activated during reading, semantic processing, generating words, and making syllable judgments. It also becomes activated during short-term memory, word retrieval and highly activated when processing the meaning of words.

Pathology & Symptoms
Because of diverse yet related functions, injury can result in a variety of disturbances depending on the area involved, including abnormalities in:
-Somesthetic and pain sensation
-The body image
-Spatial relations
-Time-sequencing motor activity
-Language
-Grammar
-Calculating numbers
-Emotion
-Attention

Attention and Visual Space
Injuries to the superior and inferior parietal lobule and the parietal-occipital junction can greatly disturb:
-Ability to make eye movements
-Maintain or shift visual attention
-Visually follow moving objects
-In the extreme result in eye paralysis

Emotion
Emotionally motivated actions can also be affected. Severe right parietal injuries in area 7

may show initial "hypokinesis" with the individual seeming very passive, inattentive, unresponsive and taking very little interest in their environment. Moreover, when an individual's symptoms are pointed out (e.g. paresis, paralysis), they may seem indifferent, or conversely, euphoric. Areas 7and 5 (and the inferior parietal lobe) receive auditory information and discern the emotional significance of this information. When the right parietal region is injured there may be difficulty differentiating forms of emotional speech.

Left Parietal Injury	Right Parietal Injury
-Minimal right sided neglect - right lobe attends to both halves of the body as well as both halves of visual space -Impact/control locating only objects within grasping/manipulation distance	-Inability to determine location, distance, spatial orientation and object size -Compromised visual abilities -Visual-spatial disorientation, clumsiness -Defective performance on line orientation tasks, maze learning, -Inability to discriminate between unfamiliar faces -Inability filter important visual information from the environment -Can result in a complete neglect of the left half of visual space Right parietal-occipital damage may also show: -Deficiency on tasks requiring detection of imbedded figures -Severe difficulty getting dressed -Easily lost/disoriented even in own home

Primary Somesthetic Receiving Areas	Somesthetic (Supplementary) Association Area
-Lessened sensory sensitivity -Lost position and pressure sense: reduced ability to detect movement of the fingers. -Inability to determine texture, shape, sequential patterning -Unable to recognize objects by touch or discriminate differences in their properties, e.g. size, texture, length, shape -Passive (non-movement) sensation less impaired. -Motor disturbances (ex: paresis with hypotnonia) -Decreased ability (or will) to initiate movement	*Mild* -Impaired movement of the hand and arm -Deficit only present when the part of the body represented is examined. *Severe* -Abnormalities in two-point discrimination -Position sense -Pressure sensitivity -Unable to determine what is held in hand. -Possible reduced ability to determine size, roughness, weight and shape properly *Laterality* -Right: bilateral abnormalities likely -Left: generally effect only the right hand

Polymodal Receiving Area	Posterior Parietal Areas 5, 7, & Supramarginal Gyrus
-Impaired Depth perception -Unable to track objects or to correctly manipulate objects in space -Decreased visual fixation -Inability to direct attention to specific objects - Impaired visual grasp/tracking -Disrupted attentional functioning *Severe* Visual neglect	-Lack of emotional responsive to pain -Indifference -Increased pain threshold -Able to tolerate pain for abnormal lengths -Failure to respond even to painful threat Secondary to tumor or seizure activity (primarily right-sided) -May instead report experiencing pain -Sensory distortions of various body parts due to abnormal parietal neocortex activation.

Inferior Parietal Lobe / Multimodal Assimilation Area
-Inability to name objects (anomia) -Agraphia -Pure word blindness -Conduction Aphasia -Lateralized time-sequencing function -Apraxias Gerstmann's Syndrome

Gerstmann's Syndrome
When the posterior left parietal lobe is injured, the ability to name objects (anomia), object and finger identification (agnosia), arithmetical abilities (acalculia), and temporal-sequential control over the hands (apraxia), and attention and neglect (particularly left sided neglect) including secondary delusional denial, disconnection, confabulation, gap filling, delusional playmates, egocentric speech are frequently compromised and collectively referred to as Gerstmann's Syndrome.

Lateralized Time-Sequencing Function
Injuries to the inferior parietal lobe can cause a disruption of visual-spatial functioning, time-sequencing ability (e.g. apraxia), as well as logic, grammar, and the capacity to perform calculations. Individuals with injuries to the inferior-parietal-occipital border of either hemisphere may have difficulty carrying out spatial-sequential tasks. For instance, when asked to draw a "square beneath a circle and a triangle beneath a square" they may draw the objects in the order described but not in proper position. This is a difficulty in conceptualizing how to place the objects in relation to one other.

Those with left inferior parietal lesions have trouble with more obvious grammar sequencing such as being unable to understand the question: "John is taller than Jim but shorter that Pete. Who is taller?" The right brain does not understand grammatical relationships, so a sentence that starts where "John" is interpreted by the right parietal area as all about "John". That is, the first word of the sentence is taken as the primary focus regardless of semantics or grammar.

If told "give me the book after you give me the pencil", the right brain responds to the order of information rather than the actual words and would present the book then the pencil.

Parietal Lobe: Activities for activation

-Judge and compare time
-Trace a maze for the first time
-Remember words and fake words
-Meaningless hand movements
-Attention exercises involving timing (e.g push a button when a light flashes)

The Temporal Lobes

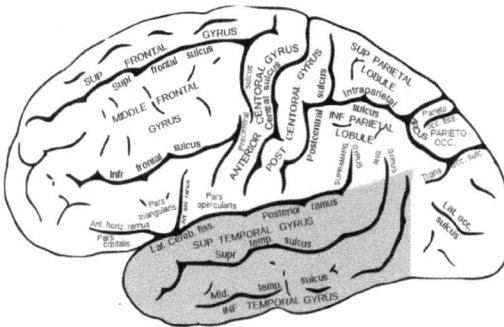

Functional Overview

The temporal lobes are unique as they are the only areas of the brain that control personalized emotional, social experience and can store and recall this information from memory. The temporal lobes also have very prominent emotional and cognitive functions, encompassing a wide range of emotional states. Much of this is in connection with the limbic system, specifically the amygdala and hippocampus with which the temporal lobes are intimately connected.

Three subdivisions can be made - superior, middle and inferior regions

The superior temporal lobe (aka the auditory neocortex)

This is the last processing and filtering of sounds before being transferred to Broca's area of the frontal lobe for responsive speaking. In this way the auditory and language areas of the brain are linked: from the amygdala, to the superior frontal lobe, to the inferior parietal lobe and to Broca's area and then back again. The signals in the superior temporal lobe have already been highly processed and analyzed Injury to the superior temporal lobe can show a number of deficits in auditory processing and association with verbal language.

The middle temporal lobe

This region processes visual input. Much of the incoming information has already been processed by older brain structures, the visual cortices. The middle temporal lobe then groups together previously processed elements into higher order units that include depth, segmenting foreground from background, and integration of information into full gestalts. An injury to this area can result in disorders called agnosias in which certain objects or types of objects cannot be perceived, processed, or there is an inability to place any meaning or memory. The right lobe is particularly strong in distinguishing speed and direction of objects.

The inferior temporal lobe

This area seems to be involved in the highest level of visual integration and contains highly developed neurons that mediate perception and recognition of specific shapes and forms. The inferior temporal lobe responds to auditory, visual and emotional stimuli. This region is particularly involved in the ability to hold focus, recognition and learning of visual discrimination, memory of objects, and spatial locations. Direction of movement, color, contrast, size, shape, orientation, and the overall processing of three-dimensionality are all processed. An injury to this area can result in visual deficits including the inability to discern and recognize faces (prosopagnosia), visual learning, and in performing visual closure in which the brain "fills in the gaps" when only part of an object is visible.

Pathology & Symptoms

Left Superior Temporal Lobe (Auditory Neocortex)	Right Superior Temporal Lobe (Auditory Neocortex)
Difficulty with: -perception of real words -word lists -numbers -backwards speech -morse code, consonants -consonant vowel syllables -nonsense syllables -transitional elements of speech -single phonemes -rhymes	Difficulty with: -acoustically related sounds -non-verbal environmental acoustics (e.g. wind, rain, animal noises) -prosodic-melodic nuances -sounds which convey emotional meaning -most aspects of music incl. temp and meter -determining location of sounds

Middle Temporal Lobe	Inferior Temporal Lobe
-Associated Visual Agnosia -Difficulty finding words -Naming deficits -Abnormalities in maintaining time order and sequence -Verbal memory impairments -Reading and naming deficits (phonological alexia) -Difficulty determining speed and direction of objects (right lobe) Those with developmental dyslexia have been found to have abnormalities here	-Difficulty in visual attention/fixation -Loss of the ability to recognize faces (prosopagnosia) -Severe disturbances involving visual discrimination learning and retention -Difficulty recognizing different shapes and patterns and objects which differ in size or color

Wernicke's Area (left Lobe)	Inferior Temporal Lobe, Amygdala, Hippocampus
"Receptive Aphasia" -Severe comprehension deficits -Difficulty with expressive speech, reading, writing, repeating, word finding, etc. -Spontaneous speech fluentcy: increased rate and may seem unable to end sentences -Incomprehensible speech -Unable to understand spoken words in their	-Memory deficits in short term emotional, visual and cognitive memory -Visual-auditory hallucinations and dream-like mental states -Temporal lobe epilepsy -Ability to sing affected (right amygdala) -Ability to properly intonate altered (right amygdala)

correct order -Cannot identify the pattern of presentation (e.g. two short and three long taps)	-Anterograde amnesia (hippocampus)

Hallucinations

Hallucinations can develop from injury to the temporal lobes. Type and intensity of the hallucinations depend on what area has been injured. Less specific auditory hallucinations such as buzzing, clicking, humming, and whispering can be associated with Heschyl's Gyrus along the transverse temporal lobe. Abnormal activity in the superior temporal lobe, particularly the right lobe, can develop musical hallucinations including a repetitious melody, singing, or individual instruments playing.

Hallucinations of single words, full sentences, comments, advice, and distant conversations that can't quite be made out are associated with either side of the superior temporal lobe. The middle and inferior temporal lobes can create visual hallucinations when damaged. The anterior inferior temporal lobe specifically tends to have the most vivid and complex forms of imagery due to its specialization in recognizing specific forms. When this abnormal activity effects the amygdala and hippocampus emotions and memories can also be evoked such as involving real people or events from memory. This includes dream-like hallucinations and the feeling of "deja vu".

With whiplash injuries, or if the skull is struck from the back or the front, the temporal lobes may hit the inside of the skull. The inferior temporal lobes are slow to mature which increases the likelihood of abnormal neural networks being formed in response to negative early life experiences. Abnormal early environmental influences such as profound traumatic stress can induce language, emotional, and memory disorders such as the repression of childhood experiences and post-traumatic stress disorder. Severe psychiatric abnormalities including schizophrenia, borderline personality disorder, and dissociative phenomenon can implicate the temporal lobes as well as the amygdala and hippocampus.

Temporal Lobe Epilepsy

Abnormal electrical activity in the temporal lobe, as in epileptic episodes, do not necessarily include involuntary movements. Someone may just seem to cease responding and stare blankly straight ahead. While this may not appear as much on the outside, internally the person may be going through a wide range of experiences or emotions. Another noteworthy cause may be severe and repeated early emotional trauma which can injure the immature hippocampus and temporal lobe, giving rise to a propensity to develop abnormal neural networks making individuals more likely to develop psychotic and severe emotional and dissociative disorders.

Automatisms – occur in 75-95% of temporal lobe seizures		
-staring -searching -groping -lip smacking -spitting -salivation	-crying -hissing -gritting/gnashing teeth -clenching fist -confused talking -screaming	-standing -running -walking -kissing -picking at one's clothes as if picking at lint

39

-laughing	-shouting	-etc.

Possible Body Sensations/Symptoms

-Numbness -Tenseness -Pressure -Heaviness -Visual sensations: things be very near or far -Feelings of strangeness or familiarity -Deja vu (~20% of cases, esp. right lobe) -Desire to be alone -Wanting something but not knowing what -Olfactory hallucinations: usually quite disagreeable and include smells like burning meat, fish, lime, acid fumes, burning feces. -There may also be digestive sensations: usually disagreeable with with bad and bitter or metallic and sour tastes	**Symptoms of possible amygdala activation** -Fear -Remembering fearful or traumatic memories -Chest or epigastric sensations -Nausea -Heart palpitations -Feelings of cold or warmth, shivering -Pallor or flushing of the face -Respiratory changes including apnea -Salivation -Belching -Farting -Sweating -Sexual arousal, feelings, or behaviors -Feelings of deja vu - the feeling of familiarity/reminiscence

Physical and Emotional Symptoms

-Laughing (gelastic epilepsy), crying (dacrystic epilepsy), and/or running seizures (cursive epilepsy) -Fear/Anxiety -Depression -Depersonalization -Pleasure -Unpleasure -Familiarity -"Out-of body experiences: often with feelings of elation, security, eternal harmony, immense joy, paradisiacal happiness, euphoria, and a "completeness"	-Sexuality changes: indiscriminate hypersexuality, public genital exposure, incestuous attempts Amygdala involvement can develop previously absent hyposexuality, hypersexuality, homosexuality, transvestism, sexual orientation confusion, or "sexual intercourse" engagement in the absence of a partner. -Religious experiences: dissociative states, feelings and hallucinogenic and dream-like recollections involving threatening men, naked women, sexual intercourse, religion, direct experience of god, demons, ghosts, etc. -Reports of communing with spirits or receiving profound otherworldly knowledge

Possible between seizure psychoses -
Range of disturbances with temporal lobe epilepsy can include:

-High rate of sexual dysfunction as well as hyposexuality	-Intensification of religious concerns -Disorders of thought

40

-Aggressiveness -Paranoia -Depression -Deepening of emotion -Intensification of religious concerns -Disorders of thought -Intensification of religious concerns -Disorders of thought	-Depersonalization -Hypergraphia -Complex visual and auditory hallucinations -Schizophrenia

Temporal Lobe: Activities for activation

-Naming/viewing pictures of new faces or experiences
-Point with hand (same side)
-Questions leading to a "yes" answer
-Read nouns aloud
-Make verb-to-noun lists
-Working with or looking at animals (left medial temporal lobe)
-Verbs/actions (left middle temporal gyrus)
-Remembering time and place (left pre-frontal cortex)
-Spatial orientation in remembered places (right hippocampus and temporal lobe)
-Listening and counting how many times a word is used in a sentence
-Performing familiar tasks
-Recall visual landmarks (spatial memory centers)
-Listen to music (opposite side ear)
-Smell stimulation (same side)
-Looking at unknown people and faces
-Remembering where an object is in the environment
-Narrative recall and list learning

The Frontal Lobes

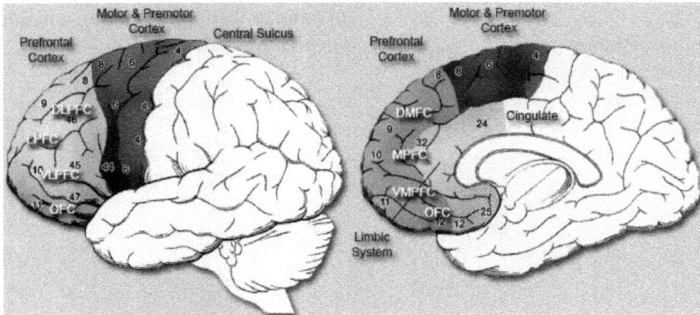

Functional Overview

The frontal lobes are the senior executive of the brain and personality. Over the course of evolution, the frontal lobes have greatly expanded in size, and are largely responsible for qualities that make us uniquely human. This includes the many achievements in art, culture, music, science, and mathematics. Although the frontal lobes are not the seat of actual intelligence, it is this area of the brain that lets humans effectively *use* our intelligence and to anticipate and plan for future possibilities. Individuals who have had (even severe) frontal lobe injury may still score normal on an IQ test as the cognitive ability remains, but may not be able to effectively put it into use.

The frontal lobes act to process, integrate, inhibit, assimilate, and remember perceptions and impulses received from the lower brain regions. Functions of the frontal lobes broadly include:
-Engaging in decision making and goal formation,
-Modulating and shapes character and personality
-Directs attention
-Maintains concentration
-Participates in information storage and memory retrieval

There are different theories about the exact essence of frontal lobe function. This includes regulating "cortical tone" with an emphasis on attention; regulating a type of "autonomy" without which the individual becomes dependent on the external environment for cues to be imitated; providing time structuring of behavior which integrates past experience with future plans; and the mediation of self-consciousness by bridging the gap between brain and mind. The frontal lobes act like an intermediary between information in and response, allowing for flexible, autonomous, and goal-directed behavior. In other animals, this tends to be much more instinctual and governed by the limbic system and brainstem.

They are also responsible for the vocalization of language including:
-Organizing in preparing to speak
-The retrieval of semantic information
-Insertion of syllables
-Temporal sequences into auditory output
-Programming and activating the primary motor areas controlling the muscles used in

vocalizing.

The right and left frontal lobes differ in their influences over arousal, attention, sexual, emotional, and memory functioning including even humor appreciation. The right hemisphere mediates emotional and melodic speech. It is dominant for arousal and appears to have bilateral inhibitory influences over arousal. The influences of the left hemisphere are more unilateral and excitatory. It mediates many aspects of speech (syntactical, lexical, semantic, and time sequencing) and is dominant over the right.

If the left frontal lobe is injured, cognitive and expressive functions tend to become suppressed and inhibited--a function not only of the injury but of the suppression of the right lobe. By contrast, right frontal injuries are more likely to give rise to disinhibitory states, including the "frontal lobe personality" discussed below.

Due to the bilateral influence of the right frontal lobe and unilateral influence of the left lobe, if unilateral left lobe damage or bilateral damage occurs the individual will express more of a depressed or apathetic affect; whereas only damage to the right lobe will more often result in an excited state. Sadness can reduce right and bi-frontal activity, though in most instances depression is directly attributed to left frontal dysfunction and reduced left frontal activity. Bilateral damage may show fluctuations between these states and thus resemble something like a bipolar tendencies.

Adults with PTSD have displayed reduced left frontal lobe activity[1]. Major brain areas involved in the pathology of PTSD are the medial frontal prefrontal cortex, anterior cingulate cortex, hippocampus and the amygdala. The amygdala controls conditioned fear responses while the medial prefrontal cortex involves the inhibition of such reactions. Injury to the medial prefrontal cortex would therefore lessen one's ability to inhibit fear. It has been theorized that frontal dysexecutive impairment due to brain injury can increase the persistence of re-experiencing trauma.[2] In schizophrenia, lateral frontal gray matter reductions and decreased brain volume and activity have been repeatedly noted.[1]

Pathology & Symptoms

Left Frontal Lobe	Right Frontal Lobe
-Depression -"Psycho-motor" stunting -Tearfulness -Apathy -Irritability -Blunted intellectual and conceptual ability -Confusion -Puerility (silliness, childishness) -Lack of environmental unawareness -Sometimes characterized as blunted form of schizophrenia	-Disinhibition: speech release, lability, and other impulsive disturbances -Mania -Confabulation (unintentional lies, false memories) -Hypersexuality -Tagentiality -Impulsive, labile, disinhibited and inappropriate social and emotional behaviors

Motor Cortex	Orbital Lobe
Supplementary Motor Area:	-Disinhibition

43

-Body may become stiff -Slow, clumsy or uncoordinated movements -Severe agraphia -Short steps and disturbances of posture, balance, and gait. -May become mute or appear catatonic **Premotor Cortex:** -Fine motor function & dexterity effected -Possible grasp reflex (i.e. stimulating the hand it will involuntarily clasp shut) **Primary Motor Area:** -Paralysis:- Initially opposite side flaccid hemiplegia then over several days muscles develop more tone and resistance to passive movements. Spasticity and hyperreflexia. Fine movements are often permanently lost.	-Hyperactive -Euphoric -Extroverted -Labile -Overtalkative -Perseveration (repetition of word or phrase) -Proneness to criminal behavior -Promiscuity -Gradiosity -Paranoia have also been observed

Broca's Area (left Lobe)	Frontal Eye Fields
-Loses the capacity to produce fluent speech -Speech becomes labored, sparse, and difficult, and may be unable to say even single words, such as "yes" or "no" -Immediately following an injury may be almost completely mute and suffer a paralysis of the upper right extremity as well as right facial weakness, unable to write, read out loud or repeat simple words	-Abnormalities in fixation -Decreased sensitivity to visual stimuli -Slowed visual scanning and searching -Inattention and Neglect -Mislocation of Sounds -Some subgroups of "schizophrenics" have been shown to suffer from smooth pursuit and sacadic abnormalities

The "Frontal Lobe Personality"
With unilateral (primarily left-sided), bilateral, or even seemingly mild frontal lobe injury individuals may display an initial waxing and waning of abnormalities, including what is referred to as the "frontal lobe personality". This may include the following symptoms:

-Tangentiality, flightiness of ideas
-Silliness or Childishness
-Impulsiveness
-Fatuous jocularity
-Lability
-Personal untidiness and dirtiness
-Poor Judgment
-Grandiosity
-Irritability, Restlessness
-Careless work habits
-Irresponsibility
-Laziness or easily tired
-Hyperexcitability
-Increased sexuality
-Promiscuity
-Extravagent money spending
-Disregard of consequences
-Tactlessness
-Changes in hunger and appetite
-Manic excitement
-Inability to produce original and imaginative thinking
-Perserveration (repetition of a particular word, phrase, or gesture)
-Compulsive use of utensils and tools (writing an endless letter with mechanical repetition of a certain phrase or word)

With significant frontal lobe pathology
-Attention may be grossly comprised
-Behavior may become fragmented
-Initiative, goal seeking, concern for consequences, planning skills, fantasy and imagination, and the general attitude toward the future may be lost
-Range of interest may shrink
-May not be able to adapt to new situations or carry out complex, purposive, and goal-directed activities
-Lack insight, judgment and common sense
-Show little to no interest in self-care or the manner in which they dress, or even if their clothes are soiled or inappropriate

A curious mixture of obsessive-compulsiveness and passive-aggressiveness may seem present. Damage to the frontal lobes, the right frontal and orbital frontal in particular, can create symptoms similar to a state of being drunk.

"Medial Frontal Lobe Syndrome"
In medial frontal lobe injury apathy is the major characteristic. Anterior cingulate gyri is primarily implicated.
-Limited speech
-Motionless (akinetic) mutism may appear - complete absence of motor activity and speech
-Transcortical motor aphasia (particularly with the left supplementary motor area)
-Lower extremity paresis and gait disturbance can be seen if damage extends to high precentral gyrus
-Sphincteric disturbance (frontal lobe incontinence). Individual tends to be indifferent to this
-Loss of spontaneity and initiative – may seem to lack "free will"

"Dorsolateral Frontal Lobe Syndrome"
This syndrome is characterized by difficulty planning new thoughts processes and carrying out sequential tasks. Although cognitive abilities such as language, memory, and visuospatial skills are themselves intact, individuals with dorsolateral injuries lack executive control and therefore cannot use these skills properly.

In this syndrome executive function deficits are paramount, they may have difficulty with:
-Planning
-Monitoring
-Flexibility of behavior
-Solving problems involving foresight, goal selection, interference resistance, use of feedback & sustained effort
-Attentiveness
-Motivation
-Perseveration
-Stimulus-bound behavior (e.g. incorrectly draws hands on clock at the 10 and 11 when asked to show 11:10)
-Echopraxia - involuntary imitation of others gestures (inhibited personal monitoring)
-Working memory may be affected and overlap with inability for sustained attention

Frontal Lobe: Activities for activation

-Generate verb-to-noun list
-Recall well-practiced material
-Meaningful hand action
-Pay attention to rhythm (Broca's area)
-Verbal exercises requiring working memory
-Cerebellar activation, esp. with hands and fingers (dentate nucleus)
Volitional eye activity or saccadic movement (opposite side)
-Interpret visual information
-Listen to complex concepts
-Learn new songs

Chapter 3
The Healing Brain

Anatomy of a brain injury
There are many different responses and health concerns that can arise from a brain injury. Some are directly from the injury itself, others are secondary results. The degree to which these occur and which they impact someone is often based on location, direction of force, and severity of the injury. The vast majority, approximately 80%, of brain injuries that are medically treated are considered "mild", while the remaining ~20% fall within the "moderate-to-severe range".

One should not be fooled by the term "mild", however. This refers ONLY to the severity AT THE TIME OF INJURY. Even if someone presents with mild initial symptoms, debilitating long-term effects can still occur. Definitions and differences between these categories are outlined in the below table. Acute symptoms following a mild brain injury (concussion) can include headaches, irritability, concentration/memory problems, sleep disturbance, dizziness, or fatigue. Approximately 43.3% of hospitalized TBI survivors are estimated to have some form of long-term disability. This risk of long-term disability increases the older the individual is when the injury occurs.

Mayo Traumatic Brain Injury Severity Classification System	
Moderate-Severe	One or more of the following criteria apply: -Death due to TBI -Loss of consciousness for 30 minutes or more -Posttraumatic anterograde amnesia of 24 hours or more -Worst Glasgow Coma Scale full score in first 24 hours <13 (unless invalidated by review) -One or more of the following: intracerebral hematoma, subdural hematoma, epidural hematoma, cerebral contusion, hemorrhagic contusion, penetrating brain trauma (dura penetrated), subarachnoid hemorrhage, brainstem injury
Mild	Does not meet the criteria for severe but presents with one or more of the following: -Loss of consciousness less than 30 minutes -Posttraumatic anterograde amnesia less than 24 hours -Skull fracture with dura intact
Symptomatic	Does not meet criteria for mild or severe but presents with one or more of the following: -Blurred vision -Confusion (mental state changes) -Dazed -Dizziness -Focal Neurological Symptoms -Headache -Nausea

Comparison of mild brain injury with moderate and severe brain injury		
Variable	**Mild Brain Injury (Concussion)**	**Moderate and Severe Brain Injury**
Clinical definition	Loss of consciousness for less than 30 minutes Alteration in consciousness or retrograde amnesia lasting less than24 hours	Loss of consciousness more than 30 minutes Posttraumatic amnesia more than 24 hours Glasgow coma scale as low as 3
Focal neurological signs	None or transient	Frequently present
Imaging (MRI, tomography)	Usually negative or very minor	Diagnostic
Natural history	Usually leads to full recovery Lack of consensus on natural history Evidence of possible prolonged sequelae	Natural history and sequelae are directly related to severity of injury and functional neuroanatomy
Predictors of persistent symptoms or disability	Consistently associated risk factors: -Psychological factors (depression, anxiety, PTSD) -Compensation and litigation -Negative expectations and beliefs	Directly related to injury characteristics
Neurocognitive testing	Often inconclusive beyond acute injury period	Essential and valuable component of ongoing clinical case
Neuronal cell damage	Metabolic and ionic effect is caused by axonal twisting or stretching can lead to secondary disconnection	Combination of cellular disruption directly related to injury and metabolic and ionic processes
Evidence of causation between injury & sequelae	Inconsistent. Debated	Not debated

Types of Injuries

Definitions of a brain injury based on cause are used to describe different types of injuries including impact force, inertial loading, penetrating and blast injuries.

Impact Injuries: Defined by the head making contact with an object and force being transferred to the brain. A rapid acceleration/ deceleration as in motor vehicle accidents with head impact, falls, and assaults can create bleeding secondary to torn blood vessels. Wider injury to the surrounding axons can also result. If this is significant it is then referred to as a *diffuse axonal injury*.

Inertial Loading Injuries: No direct contact with an object is necessary to cause a significant injury to the brain. Here the brain moves within the cranial cavity and is more likely to produce traumatic axonal injury. This can be cases of whiplash, in which the brain may sustain both "coup" (movement in the direction of the force) and "countercoup"

48

(secondary movement backward in to opposite direction of the initial force) injuries to multiple injury sites.

Penetrating Injuries: When an object passes through the protective covering of the skull, resulting in direct damage to the brain tissue. Here local tissue death becomes the primary concern.

Blast Injuries: A shock wave from an explosive device can injure the brain tissue (parenchyma) and develop brain swelling due to significant activation of microglia and astrocytes. Micrtoglia act as the first and main form of immune defense in the central nervous system, while astrocytes secrete and absorb neurotranmitters and maintain the blood-brain barrier. Blast injuries are described in more detail in chapter 5 focusing on military personnel.

Further components of an injury

Intracranial pressure and swelling
Intracranial pressure can increase after a brain injury as a result of bleeding and/or hematomas, inflammation, and swelling.

Normal intracranial pressure: 0-10mmHg
Abnormal intracranial pressure: 20mmHg or above
Associated with neurological dysfunction: 40mmHg and above
Invariably fatal: 60mmHg or above

If there is wide spread brain swelling, systemic blood pressure will increase in an attempt to maintain cerebral pressure. However, cerebral pressure can drop to such a degree that there can be oxygen loss. Neurons are particularly sensitive to this lack of blood flow and are the first type of cell to be injured. This is especially true for neurons in hippocampus, the area of the brain primarily concerned with memory, and memory problems becoming possible as a result. If there is prolonged oxygen and blood loss it will begin damaging a wide range of other cells including glial, endothelial, smooth muscle, and others.

This damage is not the direct result of oxygen loss, but rather a buildup of a substance called lactate in the tissue secondary to the lack of blood. This lactate buildup results in increased acidity (acidosis) of the pH in the local tissue. Lactic acid is produced as a normal product of cellular metabolism and generally gets removed through normal blood flow; it is only when blood flow is slowed down that build up occurs and there is tissue damage.

Brain swelling is common in cases of fatal TBI and can either impact only a small area, or it may spread and become diffuse within one hemisphere of the brain, or even spread widely throughout both hemispheres. It may be congestive, secondary to increases in blood volume, or due to edema. The majority of edema in head trauma is near the injury and causes physical disruption of the tissues, including the blood-brain barrier and loss of normal ability to regulate the blood vessels in the area.

Diffuse traumatic axonal injury contributes to at least 35% of deaths related to TBI where there are no space-occupying lesions, as well as being an important cause of severe

49

disability and vegetative states. Here forces impact small sections of axons that result in small pores or defects in the axons that over time lead to severing of the axons.

Subdural hematomas, or brain bleeds, are most often seen after a head injury, but may also develop secondary to a number of non-traumatic causes. They are estimated to happen in about 5% of head injuries. The more severe an injury, the more likely a hemotoma will occur. Most acute subdural hematomas do not form a chronic hematoma, though they may still form following a relatively mild head trauma. These are liquid and can spread in the subdural space around the brain, worsening symptoms on the affected side and a flattening of the brain region on the opposite side of the injury. As these are physical lesions which fill space withing the skull, the pressure created by them tend to cause secondary signs and symptoms.

A subarachnoid hemorrhage is relatively common following a brain injury, but rarely creates significant signs or symptoms. However, a primary traumatic subarachnoid hemorrhage (such as caused by a punch just under the mandible) can rupture the vertebral or basilar arteries and carries a high risk of mortality.

Intracerebral hemorrhages are most often seen in the frontal and temporal lobes. Superficial bleeds are most often due to extensive cuts and scrapes while deeper hematomas tend to occur when there is greater force such as high velocity vehicle accidents.

Following a traumatic brain injury, the body quickly begins a series of secondary processes that collectively contribute to cell injury and/or repair. These secondary events often create long-term neurological symptoms, including cognitive dysfunction. These early events can be divided into three periods: those which arise within minutes after an injury, those that evolve over the first 24 hours, and events that may be more delayed in onset, appearing between 24 and 72 hours post-injury.

Initiation of Acute Secondary Events Following Brain Injury	
Within minutes	Cell/axon stretching, compaction of neurofilaments, impaired axonal transport, axonal swelling, axonal disconnection
	Blood–brain barrier disruption
	Excessive neuronal activity: Glutamate release
	Widespread neurotransmitter changes: Catecholamines, serotonin, histamine, GABA, acetylcholine
	Hemorrhage (heme, iron-mediated toxicity)
	Seizures
	Physiologic disturbances: Decreased cerebral blood flow, hypotension, hypoxemia, increased intracranial pressure, decreased cerebral perfusion pressure
	Increased free radical production
	Disruption of calcium homeostasis
	Mitochondrial disturbances
Minutes–24 hr	Oxidative damage: Increased reactive oxygen and nitrogen species (lipid peroxidation, protein oxidation, peroxynitrite), reduction in endogenous antioxidants (e.g., glutathione)
	Ischemia

	Initiation of Acute Secondary Events Following Brain Injury
	Edema
	Enzymatic activation (kallikrein-kinins, calpains, caspases, endonucleases, metalloproteinases)
	Decreased ATP: Changes in brain metabolism (altered glucose utilization and switch to alternative fuels), elevated lactate
	Cytoskeleton changes in cell
	Widespread changes in gene expression: cell cycle, metabolism, inflammation, receptors, channels and transporters, signal transduction, cytoskeleton, membrane proteins, neuropeptides, growth factors, and proteins involved in transcription/translation
	Inflammation: Cytokines, chemokines, cell adhesion molecules, influx of leukocytes, activation of resident macrophages
24–72 hr	Non-ischemic metabolic failure

The body's healing response to an injury

Neurons in the brain are continuously receiving, processing, and integrating information from the entire body, including the brain, to then send out signals to other neurons and cells throughout the body. Brain injury affects neuronal circuitry by causing the death of neurons and glial cells (described below) and destroying the connections between them. This includes the dendrites and axons through which neurons receive and emit signals and neurotransmitters.

Brain injury often leads to excessive accumulation of neurotransmitters in the brain tissue. In particular glutamate, and excitatory neurotransmitter, can overstimulate neurons and cause further cell death. The brain works to limit the spread of damage by forming a glial scar that seals off the damaged region. Glial cells (astrocytes, oligodendrocytes, and microglia) are particularly important in this process.

Astrocytes act in a protective way to produce glucose and other nutrients while supporting the viability of the surviving cells. Astrocytes were once considered just the glue filling the space between neurons, and have long been recognized for their importance in maintaining brain environment stability (homeostasis), providing nutrition for neurons, and recycling neurotransmitters. More recently, they have been shown to control blood flow, functional control of synapses, and processes of plasticity and regeneration.

Brain injury leads to increased neural plasticity, the brain's ability to adapt, in the unaffected regions. This acts to allow neurons in these areas to take over sensory or motor functions that had been performed by the damaged areas. This is a critical function of the recovery process. Neural plasticity peaks within one to three months after injury; this creates a unique window of opportunity. During this window, neurorehabilitation is most effective. However, significant improvements can occur even at later stages.

Astrocytes become activated after events such as neurological trauma and stroke. This phenomenon, known as reactive gliosis, is accompanied by an altered expression of many genes and profound changes in the properties and function of astrocytes. The cellular hallmarks of reactive gliosis are the thickening (hypertrophy) of astrocyte processes, proliferation of more astrocytes, and increases in the amount of intermediate cellular filaments (also called nanofilaments). Intermediate filaments form a scaffold-like network within the cell cytoplasm, a highly dynamic structure involved in cell signaling, scarring, and migration, that can act as a signaling platform. This helps cells and tissues cope with stress in both health and recovery.

The capacity for astrocytes to take up and use the inhibitory neurotransmitter GABA is reduced in the area surrounding brain cells affected by injury. The inhibition of neurons by excessive GABA directly counteracts neural plasticity and impairs functional recovery.

The Role of the Immune System
The immune system in the brain itself, along with immune cells and molecules from the blood play an important role in the normal development of nervous tissue. It is also pivotal in the brain and spinal cord's response to injuries. Reactive cells in the glial scar produce molecules that inhibit the growth of neuronal processes and limit recovery. At a later stage (weeks after injury and beyond), when the activity of these cells are no longer needed for limiting the spreading of tissue damage, the immune system signals the astroglial cells in the scar to reduce their activation. This is necessary for repair and functional recovery to be effective.

The innate immune response is the rapid first line of defense against infection. It lacks specificity and responds in the same manner to a wide range of triggering events. In contrast, the adaptive immune response is inefficient at the time of injury with an infectious agent (such as a virus or bacteria), but its efficiency increases with time. The adaptive immune response is very specific and has "memory,"—it responds in a much more rapid and efficient manner upon a repeated encounter with the same bacteria or virus. Both the innate and adaptive immune systems rely on many different immune cell types to operate.

Innate immune response cells called microglia constantly survey brain tissue for protein buildups or cellular debris, which they efficiently remove. However, their prolonged and excessive activity is associated with a release of substances that are toxic to neurons. Monocytes recruited from the blood are important regulators of the local immune response, including the activity of microglia.

The complement system, a group of immune system proteins that initiate inflammation and eliminate pathogenic bacteria, has multiple roles in the central nervous system. During normal development, this system is involved in eliminating excessive synapses. The same process in adulthood, however, can be the first step in neurodegeneration. The complement system also functions as a regulator of neurogenesis in a healthy brain and after ischemic stroke. Because of this, in the diseased or injured brain, the complement system can either increase tissue damage or can be protective and contribute to repair and recovery.

Immune system activity declines as we age, and the resulting imbalance could be one reason for poorer recovery from brain injury in older individuals and for the age-related decline of perception, motor behavior, cognition, and memory function.

Chapter 4
Brain Injury in Children and Adolescents

According to the Center of Disease Control, traumatic brain injury is the leading cause of death and acquired disability in children and teens in the United States. The two largest at-risk groups are those 0-4 years and adolescents ages 15-19. In children ages 0-15, there are almost half a million head injury emergency room visits each year. 80-90% of these are considered mild, 7-8% considered moderate, and 5-8% are considered severe.

Most cases in those 0-4 years old are due to falls. These young children are however also more susceptible to abusive head trauma (AHT), previously known as shaken baby syndrome. Older children and teens are more likely to sustain a concussion as a result of sport injuries, falls, being struck by something, or motor vehicle accidents.

Outcomes of recovery are dependent on many factors including severity, time of injury, and the developmental state of the brain at the time of injury. Evidence shows that young children are just, if not more, susceptible to the effects of a brain injury than older children. There is a higher likelihood of diffuse injury and brain swelling (44%) compared to adults. Post-traumatic seizures are particularly relevant, as occurrence within the first week is twice as likely (10% vs. 5%) to occur compared to adults.

New Psychiatric Disorders
There has been a recorded 54-63% occurrence of new psychiatric disorders in children with severe TBI and 10-21% in children with mild or moderate TBI 2 years after injury.

Predictors of these developing include:
-Severity of the injury
-Preinjury psychiatric disorders
-Preinjury family function
-Family psychiatric history
-Socioeconomic status
-Preinjury intellectual function
-Preinjury adaptive function.

The most consistent of these was preinjury and postinjury family function including family burden and family distress.

Psychiatric Disturbances Following Brain Injury

Disturbance	Associated Regions	Other Factors
Attention-deficit/ hyperactivity disorder	Right putamen, thalamus, orbital frontal gyrus	-Preinjury family functioning -Not associated with injury severity, family function, socioeconomic status, family stressors, family psychiatric history, gender or injured area

Personality changes	Superior frontal gyrus, frontal white matter	-Affective instability, agression, disinhibition, apathy, paranoia ~40% incidence in severe injury -Often with adaptive and intellectual imparments
Post-Traumatic Stress Disorder (reexperiencing)	Right limbic area (including cingulum) lower lesion fraction	-Injury severity, socioeconomic status, and mood or anxiety disorder at time of injury
Post-Traumatic Stress Disorder (hyperarousal)	Left temporal lesions and lower frequency of orbitofrontal lesions	-Injury severity, socioeconomic status, and mood or anxiety disorder at time of injury
Obsessions	Mesial prefrontal and temporal lesions	-Psychosocial adversity, higher prevalence in females
Obsessive-Compulsive Disorder	Frontal and temporal lobes	-Psychosocial adversity, higher prevalence in females
Anxiety Disorder	Superior frontal gyrus, frontal white matter	-May include overanxious disorder, specific phobia, separation anxiety disorder, avoidant disorder -Associated with preinjury anxiety symptoms and younger age at time of injury
Mania/hypomania	Frontal and temporal lobes	-Injury severity, family history of major mood disorders

Neurocognitive Development and Arrest
Children's brains are still developing and continue to generally go through significant spikes of maturing through the age of about 22. During these peaks new neural connections increase dramatically in particular brain regions and throughout the brain. The age, developmental stage of the child, and location of injury can delay or arrest further development or the learning of new skills. This has been referred to as "neurocognitive stall"[4]. Peak development ages have been shown to occur at approximately 0-1 years, 3-5 years, 7-10 years, 14-15 years, 17-19 years and lastly around 21-22 years of age.

The time between birth and about 5 years old is when the developing brain forms the most new neural pathways and connections. For this reason, young children who suffer a brain injury in this age range tend to have poorer overall outcomes. During this time the most apparent development occurs in the lower brain functions of the brain stem and cerebellum as well as the limbic system associated with normal emotional development.

Due to the progressive development of brain regions, preschoolers who sustain a frontal lobe injury will often appear unaffected shortly after the injury. As they age however, and frontal lobe functions become more prominent in their conscious state and cognitive functioning, the injured area may not develop or function properly. This can result in long-term psychosocial and behavioral problems along with serious learning, behavioral and emotional problems as the child grows older. This can be misconstrued or misdiagnosed as a learning disability or a behavioral disorder rather than the effect of an injury to the brain.

Ages 3-5 years
All regions of the brain undergo rapid neural growth in visuospatial, visuo-auditory, and executive functions. Here the child refines skills in forming images, using words, placing things in a particular order, and problem solving. The sensory motor region of the brain peaks about age 6-7 as rationale, logic, and mathematical thinking become more available.

Ages 7-10 years
The frontal executive functions begin to rapidly accelerate in development. This involves further visuo-spatial functioning and visuo-auditory regions. By age 10 the child is generally suited to perform formal operations such as calculations and the perception and placement of meaning to familiar objects.

Ages 14-15 years
The visuo-auditory, visuospatial, and sensory systems tend to reach their peak within a 1 year interval of one another. The ability to review information and operations, find flaws within them, and create new ones develops. At this time social development and the establishment of a firm peer system outside of the family structure also becomes more important to them as self-identity is explored and developed.

Ages 17-19 years
The young individual tends to begin questioning information they are given, will reconsider it based on experience, and form a new concept when necessary while incorporating their own ideas. This tends to continue until the mid-twenties sometime when mylenation of the frontal cortex becomes complete.

In the context of the eight circuit model of consciousness, as explored in my previous book *Circuits and Shen: Models of the Evolution of Consciousness and Chinese Medicine,* these age ranges roughly correlate to the bio-survival (0-2 years), emotional-territorial (2-5 years), neuro-semantic (7-10 years), and the socio-sexual circuits (12-19 years). Below is a simplified reference of the "lower" four circuits. The "higher" four circuits can also come into play with certain mental-emotional concerns following a brain injury such as mania and schizophrenia. For a more thorough investigation of these concepts and treatment approaches refer to *Circuits and Shen.*

First Four Circuits of Consciousness		
Circuit	**Approximate Age Of Standard Development**	**Developmental Attributes**
Bio-survival	0-2 years	Basic survival mechanisms, ability to thrive, eating, sleeping, digestion, nurturing bond, undifferentiated from everything else particular primary nurturing figure, fear *imprint:* safety (approach) vs danger (avoidance) *neural connections most active:* brainstem, cerebellum, insula
Emotional-Territorial	2-5 years	Establishment of boundaries between self and external world, learning to control and manipulate the world, basic reproductive drives, tantrums, anger, lack of empathy for others, narcissism *imprint:* dominance vs submissiveness *neural connections most active:* limbic system, amygdala
Neuro-semantic	7-10 years	Formal operations, problem-solving, map making, linear rationale, mathematics, organization and list making, logic and "left-brained" thinking *imprint:* intellectualism and rationality *neural connections most active:* parietal, frontal lobes
Socio-sexual	12-19 years	Social and peer support groups, separation from family unit and further ego establishment, sexuality, charisma, conformity and upholding societal morals and norms *imprint:* social and sexual intelligence and roles *neural connections most active:* prefrontal lobes

Causes of Pediatric and Adolescent Brain Injury

Non-traumatic
- Brain tumors
- Anoxia/hypoxia
- Infections
- Stroke
- Toxic substance/environmental exposure

Abusive Head Trauma (AHT, previously known as Shaken Baby Syndrome)
-Often committed by a frustrated caregiver or parent in response to crying, temper tantrums or issues with developmental milestones such as toilet training. If an infant is violently shaken, the head sustains multiple impacts of coup and countercoup injuries.
- Most common in infants 0-5 years of age.
-Accounts for an estimated 50-80% of head-trauma related deaths in those under 2 years old
-Study of 10,555 survivors showed 77% were under 1 year of age (60% male, 40% female)
-Higher risk in infants with excessive crying from birth-4 months

-71% of individuals responsible were male caregivers (in those who admitted the abuse) – 56% being biological fathers, 16% being a mothers boyfriend, 15% was the child's biological mother. Because of this familial tendency it is important to assess risk of continued abuse and provide information, resources, and support connections.

Diagnostics: medical professionals look for
        -Subdural hemorrhage or hermatoma:
        -Cerebral edema
        -Retinal hemorrhage: present in 85% of AHT/SBS

Prognosis
70-85% survive with long-term disabilities such as behavioral problems, learning disabilities, blindness, deafness, seizures and cerebral palsy. 15-30% cases are fatal.

Concussion and Mild Brain Injury
Hundreds of thousands of teen athletes each year are suspected of experiencing a concussion. While most of these are mild, making a complete recovery, approximately 10% of these athletes will have persistent symptoms including problems with:
-Attention
-Memory
-Fatigue
-Sleep
-Headaches
-Dizziness
-Irritability
-Personality changes

When these symptoms become chronic and persist it is referred to as Post-Concussion Syndrome (PCS). This can cause difficulties in their performance in school as well as sports. School, family, and social life can all be impacted as a result.

If they continue their athletics too soon without allowing for a full recovery they can experience what is known as "Second impact syndrome" which can be fatal or cause severe disability as a result of brain swelling or bleeding. Another risk of secondary impact is Chronic Traumatic Encephalopathy (CTE), a progressive degenerative disease which includes dementia, memory loss, aggression, confusion, and depression. While CTE appears similar to Alzheimer's Disease in symptoms, they differ in the disease process. CTE has been demonstrated to stem from structural changes in the brain tissue including a unique buildup of abnormal Tau proteins.

Fortunately, in recent years, awareness of the impact of concussions on youth have resulted in increased education of teachers, coaches, and parents. As of 2015 all 50 states had enacted concussion laws governing youth sports, most of which contain guidelines on how to approach a suspected concussion and when to remove a player until evaluated by a medical professional. This is because rest and recovery are essential. This may include staying home from school for a period of time while restricting time spent text messaging, playing video games, or using a computer/smart phone for extended periods of time.

Educational Need Considerations

Some children who have had a brain injury will require special accommodations in their educational environment. At times these are basic interventions in the classroom. Others may need a formal plan put into place. This is referred to as a 504 Accommodation Plan where a specially designed individual approach to their education is formed. Public schools are federally mandated to provide a free appropriate public education through special education supports and services, also called Specialized Academic Instruction (SAI), to children with eligible disabilities.

The 504 Accommodation Plan is intended to eliminate discrimination against students with disabilities and may address possible options such as:
-Preferential seating
-Extended time on tests or assignments
-Tests given in a quiet or alternate setting
-Word banks being provided during tests
-Additional rest breaks
-Shortened assignments
-Visual aids
-Books on CD or text-to-speech software

Areas of Possible Impairment Impacting Education	
Motor Impairments	Gross and fine motor, strength, coordination, speed Rigidity, tremors, spasticity, ataxia, apraxia
Physical Effects	Disruption in growth, eating disorders, development of diabetes, thermal dysregulation
Feeding	Dysphagia (difficulty swallowing)
Sensory Impairments	Vision, hearing, difficulty with worksheets, completion of only half of an assignment sheet due to visual neglect, disorientation, slow to produce written material
Communication Impairments	Expressive and receptive movement, taking turns in conversation, inability to summarize/articulate thoughts, talking around a subject, difficulty or inability to understand metaphors and figurative speech, difficulty finding words
Cognitive Impairments	Attention: easily distracted, delayed response to questions, difficulty staying on topic, unable to complete task without prompting, blurts out answers inappropriately, fatigued by mid-afternoon
	Memory: remembering assignments/materials, learning routines, homework tasks, unable to recall content of material, difficulty remembering 2-3 step directions, repeated exposure needed
	Executive Functioning/Higher Learning: difficulty with organization and completion of long term assignments, unable put together necessary steps to reach goal, unable to problem solve as issues arise, difficulty drawing conclusions from facts, difficulty evaluating and altering performance
Academic	Learning difficulties, inability to take notes while listening, difficulty

	copying information from board
Fatigue	Physical and cognitive
Medical Issues	Seizures, headache, pain, orthopedic issues
Social-emotional or behavioral difficulties	Irritability/easily frustrated, disinhibition, socially inappropriate actions or words, mood swings, difficulty fitting in with peers, easily misled by peer pressure, misperception of social cues or interactions, impulsivity to leave seat/classroom, lack of awareness/denial of impairments, appears unmotivated, withdrawal, depression, apathy
Family difficulties	Difficulty interacting, stress upon family, abuse, neglect or needs not being met at home
Post-school Concerns	Vocational issues, housing issues

Fewer than 2% of children 0-19 years old with a brain injury are referred for special education programs, placing the onus on public schools to ensure the child's education. One study found that close to 60% of children with a TBI fail to receive any school-based services due to delayed effects and a failure to recognize a need for continued monitoring. This can make the schooling process quite difficult and frustrating for the individual.

Possible Instructional and Compensatory Strategies	
Attention and concentration	-Clear learning objectives -Short, concise instructions -Shorten assignments; divide work into small sections -Minimize distractions -Non-verbal attention cues -Additional breaks -Reward on-task behavior
Memory and Learning Processing	-Learning objectives for each lesson -Link new information to relevant prior knowledge -"My turn, our turn, your turn" teaching method (modeling, guided practice, independent practice) -Hands-on learning opportunities -Frequent repetition and summation of information -Utilization and education in using graphic organizers -Memory devices -Extra set of books for home -Direct Instruction Curriculum materials
Organization	-Templates for assignments, projects, papers -Visual schedule -Assistance with homework planner, backpack check -Assignments and notes provided on school website -Utilize different colored notebooks for each subject -Break long-term projects into specific timelines for each part
Following Directions	-Oral and written instruction

	-Highlight written instruction -Task-analyze directions into simple steps
Auditory-Perceptual	-Limit amount of information presented -Speak at a slower pace, with pauses -Provide visuals to accompany verbal information -Use a peer to repeat oral instructions
Visual-Perceptual	-Limit amount of information on page -Use large print -Present materials on a slant -Longer viewing times -Seating close to front of classroom -Arrows or cue words for orientation -Maps or teach student to navigate schedule
Motor-Physical	-Assistive technology and adapted devices to provide access -Allow extra time for tasks and changing classes -Adapted physical education

Related Services for Children and Adolescents
-Speech-language pathology
-Auditology services
-Interpreting services
-Psychological services
-Physical therapy
-Occupational therapy
-Acupuncture and Naturopathic approaches
-Recreation, including therapeutic recreation
-Early identification and assessment of disabilities in children
-Counseling services, rehabilitative counseling
-Orientation and mobility services (for visual impairment)
-Medical services for diagnostics or evaluation
-School health and nursing services
-Social work services in schools
-Parent counseling and training

Resources:

BrainSTEPS (Strategies Teaching Educators, Parents and Students) Child and Adolescent Brain Injury School Re-entry Program.
www.brainsteps.net

Lash & Associates Publishing/Training Inc – educational books, DVDS, and tip cards
www.lapublishing.com

Project Optimal Traumatic Brain Injury Program – online self-study program providing advanced, specialized training for education specialists
www.innovative-learning.com/projectoptimal/?pg=traumatic-brain-injury

Blosser JL, DePompei R. Pediatric Traumatic Brain Injury: Proactive Intervention. 2nd ed. Clifton Park, NY: Delmar Learning; 2003.

DePompei, R, Blosser J, Savage R, Lash M. Back to School After Mild Brain Injury or Concussion. Youngsville, NC: Lash and Associates Publishing/Training, Inc.; 2011

Lash M, Wolcott G, Pearson S. Signs and Strategies for Educating Students with Brain Injuries. Wake Forest, NC: Lash and Associates Publishing/Training, Inc.; 2005

Lebby PC, Asbell SJ. The Source for Traumatic Brain Injury: Children and Adolescents. East Moline, IL: LinguiSystems; 2007.

Max JE, Ibahim F, Levin H: Neuropsychological and psychiatric outcomes of traumatic brain injury in children. Cognitive and Behavioral Abnormalities of Pediatric Diseases. Edited by Nass, R, Frank Y. New York. Oxford University Press. 2010

Savage R, Wolcott G. Educational Dimensions of Acquired Brain Injury. Austin, TX: Pro-Ed; 1994.

Ylvisaker, M. Traumatic Brain Injury Rehabilitation: Children and Adolescents. 2nd ed. Boston, MA: Butterworth, Heineman; 1998.

Chapter 5
Brain Injuries in the Military

The Department of Defense (DoD) did not begin surveying traumatic brain injury until 2006. Between this time and 2012 over 229,000 service members were diagnosed with traumatic brain injury (TBI). 22% of those returning from Operation Iraqi Freedom (OIF) were reported to have at least one. Most of these cases were mild, with a full recovery expected, with 8% expected to have persistent symptoms. Certain Military Occupational Specialties (MOS) within the military run a higher risk of sustaining a TBI, including infantry, Explosive Ordinance Device (EOD) personnel and special forces. Outside of field operations, injuries to the brain can occur in training accidents such as rappelling, shooting, parachuting, other specialty activities, or from operating within closed-in spaces such as tanks or submarines.

55% of combat injuries were found to be related to blast injuries, 27% were found to be from "multiple mechanisms" and 7% the result of vehicular injuries. Those who experienced penetrating injuries are at a higher risk for severe complications than those who sustained a blunt TBI. 43% of those with TBI had a psychiatric disorder noted in their records, with PTSD being the most common. For more details of PTSD refer to chapter 31.

The differences in the military healthcare system from the civilian system creates different approaches to diagnostic and treatment approaches. The complexity of the DoD and VA healthcare systems, and the high prevalence of compounded symptoms such as PTSD can make the recovery process particularly challenging. Creating a supportive environment of people who can understand the challenges of service members as they struggle with conflicting feelings about their combat experience, military status, and their injuries is critical for the healing process. This can include a wide range of support from family members, healthcare providers, therapists, and peer counselors.

Blast Injuries
Blast injuries, or blast-induced neurotrauma (BINT), is a common mechanism of injury in recent wars and often referred to as the signature wound of Operation Iraqi Freedom (OIF) and Operation Enduring Freedom (OEF). These accounted for nearly 55% of combat injuries including from IEDs, rocket-propelled grenades, mortars, mines, bombs and grenades. In most cases this involves a combination of both blunt and blast injuries

Concussive blasts can impact the body at a velocity beyond the speed of sound. This is quickly followed by a very high-velocity wind capable of being deadly. Individuals positioned between a blast and a building often suffer from injuries two to three times the degree of injury of a person in an open space as explosions near or within hard solid surfaces become amplified by two to nine times due to shockwave reflection.

Blast exposure has been reported to cause brain edema and considerable metabolic disturbances in the brain including significantly decreased glucose, magnesium, and ATP concentrations; increased lactate concentration, and impaired sodium and potassium function which is essential for neural signaling. Oxidative stress, changes in antioxidant–enzyme defense systems, and later cognitive deficits have also been seen.

63

Evidence is accumulating that a primary blast injury also affects organs organs that contain fluid such as the lungs and liver, allowing for the transfer of the huge amount of kinetic energy and sudden pressure increases. This can result in symptoms such as:
-Apnea
-Rapid breathing
-Slow heart rate (bradycardia)
-Hypotension
-Dilatation of the peripheral blood vessels that results in lowered blood pressure
These are frequently seen immediately after blast exposure and may increase risk of complications.

Prevention of these injury types prove difficult as body armor, while protecting from shrapnel and penetrating injuries (secondary and tertiary blast injuries) and undoubtedly creating better survival rates, actually acts as an improved contact surface for energy transfer. It also serves as a reflecting surface that concentrates the power of an explosion as the blast wave resonates internally. [1]

Hierarchy of Blast Related Injuries	
Primary Blast Injury	Direct impact to the body of blast force
Secondary Blast Injury	Injury due to energized debris (projected or falling) or shrapnel
Tertiary Blast Injury	The displaced body impacts the ground, wall, or other object
Quarternary Blast Injury	Inhalation of gases or other toxic substances

Diagnostics/Assessment
In 2006 the Defense and Veterans Brain Injury Center (DVBIC) developed an operational definition of traumatic brain injury in military operations. It is stated as " an injury to the brain resulting from an external force and/or acceleration/deceleration mechanism from an event such as a blast, fall, direct impact, or motor vehicle accident which causes an alteration of mental status typically resulting in the temporally related onset of symptoms such as: headache, nausea, vomiting, dizziness/balance problems, fatigue, trouble sleeping, sleep disturbances, drowsiness, sensitivity to light/noise, blurred vision, difficulty remembering, and/or difficulty concentrating".

Various testing protocols were developed including:
-Military Acute Concussion Evaluation (MACE)
-Standardized Assessment of Concussion (SAC): assesses four cognitive domains: orientation, immediate memory, concentration, memory recall
-Brief Traumatic Brain Injury Screen (BTBIS)
-Combat stress screening
-Neuropsychological Assessment (20 minute assessment required for any service member preparing for deployment)

-Neurobehavioral Symptom Inventory (NSI): able to assess most common TBI
    symptoms
-State-Trait Anxiety Inventory (STAI): mood and sleep scale
-Automated Neuropsychological Assessment Metrics (ANAM): mood and sleep
    scale
-ANAM Simple Reaction Time and Continuous Performance subtests: objective
    assessment of cognitive performance
-Repeatable Battery for the Assessment of Neuropsychological Status

Stateside screening occurs through Post-Deployment Health Assessment (PDHA) and Post-Deployment Health Reassessment (PDHRA)

Standard Treatment Methods
According to Clinical Practice Guidelines (CPG) in deployment settings
-Symptom Management: pharmacological intervention, glasses, etc.
-Education: educational materials, flyers, national website
-Implementation of duty restrictions
-MEDEVAC to hospital or continental United States as necessary

Levels of medical care	
Level I	Other service members in field, Battalion Aid Stations (BAS): observation, rest, non-critical symptom management
Level II	Mobile, basic medical care, basic diagnostics, holding limited to 72 hours
Level III	Combat Support Hospital: highest in-field care. Full surgical and intensive care capabilities, CT scans and diagnostics
Level IV	Non-battlefield facilities such as Landstuhl Regional Medical Center in Germany, MRI, neurology evaluation
Level V	Stateside facilities comparable to level I trauma centers

Stateside treatment is through primary care according to VA-DoD concussion management guidelines. Those with severe or penetrating injuries are managed according to civilian TBI guideline.

-VA Polytrauma System of Care (PSC) -team develops individual follow-up plans for each veteran after discharge
-Case workers, clinical psychologists, neuropsychologists, social workers, etc.
-Civilian partnership programs for model community reintegration may be sought and can be helpful
-Community Integrated Rehabilitation (CIR): e.g. DVBIC (Defense and Veterans Brain Injury Center), Residential Community Programs, Comprehensive holistic day treatments, Home-based Programs

Medical Evaluation and Discharge
When a service member has experienced a TBI which renders them unable to perform required duties they may be retired from the military under a medical discharge. This process involves evaluation by both the Medical Evaluation Board (MEB) and the Physical Evaluation Board (PEB). The MEB first determines whether the service member's long-

term medical condition allows them to continue to meet medical retention standards as well as having military physicians clearly document medical conditions and limitations that may exist as a result. These findings are considered informal and are then referred to the PEB who will formally determine if one is fit to continue service and eligibility for disability compensation. The PEB will recommend one of the following:
-Return to duty (with or without assignment limitations)
-Be placed on the temporary disabled/retired list (TDRL)
-Separation from active duty
-Medical retirement
If medical retirement is determined, the PEB rates the disability on a scale 0-100% scale in increments of 10% according to the VA Schedule for Rating Disabilities.

Emotional Impact of Unit Separation and Peer Support
Removal from one's unit or cohort can often increase anxiety and the likelihood of PTSD. Medical evacuation removes the service member from their primary support system as well as bringing on feelings of guilt about abandoning their brothers and sisters in arms. For this reason many service members will not report or present for medical attention and opt to "tough it out". This increases the overall likelihood of medical errors, subsequent injury and possible psychological distress should post-concussion syndrome develop.

Concerns upon Returning Home
As with any brain injury case, one's family life can be greatly impacted following an injury. A service member may or may not be able to participate in discussions and decisions in their medical treatment and recovery expectations. Family members may have to suddenly adjust to the service member experiencing symptoms that can range from mild memory impairment to being minimally responsive and bed bound. The service member may have difficulty successfully engaging in treatment due to a tendency to forget appointments, forget to take medications, the inability to drive to a doctor's office, or general confusion. This can often be a complex process of adapting, coping and grieving.

Resources:
Veterans Crisis line: 1-800-273-8255 Press 1

Defense and Veterans Brain Injury Center
www.dvbic.org

Defense Center for Excellence for Psychological Health and TBI
www.dcoe.health.mil

US Air Force of Excellence for Medical Multimedia: TBI
www.traumaticbraininjuryatoz.org

Mental Wellness Program including TBI Issues for Post-deployment
www.dvbic.org/service-members---veterans/care-coordination.aspx

Brainline.org
www.brainline.org

National Intrepid Center of Excellence
www.dcoe.health.mil/ComponentCenters/NICoE.aspx

Military TBI Care Coordination Program
www.dvbic.org/service-members---veterans/care-coordination.aspx

Overview of VA TBI Rehabilitation Programs
www.polytrauma.va.gov/understanding-tbi/recovery-and-rehabilitation/rehabilitation-programs

Returning Veterans Project (Oregon/Washington)
www.returningveterans.org/resources

Part 2

Treatment Approaches

Chapter 6
Diet and Exercise

Chemical disruptions that result from a head injury can alter metabolism within the brain. There may be an increase in extracellular potassium and glutamate, which in turn increases calcium. Glucose uptake, which is what the brain uses as energy to function, increases within 8 days of the injury in order to meet the new increased energy needs of reestablishing a balanced functioning. This is followed by a long period of decreased glucose metabolism. The magnitude and duration of this depression increases with severity and age of injury. Increases in reactive oxygen species (ROS) and related DNA damage cause further problems in glucose processing and thus brain function.[1]

Select diets and exercise can help regulate molecules important for neural plasticity, such as brain-derived neurotrophic factor (BDNF). This affects normal function and recovery following an injury to the brain. BDNF is a regulator of survival, growth and differentiation in neurons during development. It is now known that BDNF works to translate activity into synaptic and cognitive plasticity, as well as being able to affect neurotransmitter release, stimulate proteins synthesis, and regulate DNA/RNA transcription factors. If BDNF is blocked, it has been shown to impair learning and memory in rats. BDNF, but not nerve growth factor (NGF) seems to play a role in consolidating long-term memories as well. [2, 3]

Exercise and Neural Repair
Physical activity is thought to benefit neuronal function by increasing brain-derived neurotrophic factor (BDNF) levels and reducing oxidative stress. Specifically, exercise has been found to be important in regulating neurite development [81] , maintenance of the synaptic structure [82], axonal elongation [83], and neurogenesis [84] in the adult brain. Physical activity displays long-lasting changes in structure and function of the nervous system, suggesting that regular exercise can lead to a brain that is more resistant to injury. 30 minutes of physical activity has been shown to elevate one's serotonin levels.

Exercise after an injury seems promising in helping to facilitate recovery, though more studies are necessary as to determine when, and to what extent it should be integrated. Exercise applied after experimental traumatic brain injury has been shown to have beneficial effects, but the effects seem to depend on the resting period post-injury and the severity of the injury. [85] It has been demonstrated that different types of exercise seem to stimulate different brain regions.[1] While preliminary, these are outlined in the table below:

Exercise type	Brain Region	Functions
Aerobic Exercise	Hippocampus	Memory
Sports Drills	Prefrontal cortex/basal ganglia	Attention, multitasking, inhibition
Yoga	Frontal lobe, insula	Thought & emotion integration
Weight lifting	Prefrontal cortex	Complex thinking, problem-solving, multitasking

High intensity intervals	Hypothalamus	Appetite regulation

Diet

General Food Considerations For Brain Health

-Leafy greens: Kale, romaine lettuce, swiss chard
-Spinach
-Beets
-Sweet potato
-Cauliflower, broccoli
-Avacado
-Coconut oil
-Dark chocolate
-Blueberries
-Bone broth
-Egg yolk
-Extra virgin olive oil
-Nuts: walnuts
-Beans
-Rosemary

Daily Nutrient Recommendations

Dr. Kedar Prasad, Ph.D. has formulated nutritional protocols for situations involving maintaning brain health, prevention of concussions among professional athletes, prevention of secondary brain injuries, and nutritional needs following a brain injury. These are outlined in the table below:

	Concussion Prevention (professional athlete)	Secondary Brain Injury Prevention	Following Brain Injury
Vitamin A		3,000 IU	5,000 IU
Natural Vitamin E	3,000 IU	400 IU	400 IU
Vitamin C	400 IU	1,000 mg	2,000 mg
Vitamin D3	1,000 mg	1,000 UI	1,000 mg
Vitamin B1 (Thiamine)	1,000 IU	10 mg	10 mg
Vitamin B2 (Riboflavin)	10 mg	4 mg	5 mg
Vitamin B3 (Nicotinamide)	4 mg	100 mg	150 mg
Vitamin B6 (Pyroxine)	400 mcg	4 mg	4 mg
Folic Acid	100 mcg	800 mcg	400 mcg
Vitamin B12	200 mcg	100 mcg	150 mcg

(cobalamin)			
Biotin	15 mg	150 mcg	200 mg
Pantothenic Acid	5 mg	15 mg	10 mg
Zinc glycinate	100 mcg	5 mg	15 mg
Selenium	Proprietary amount	100 mcg	200 mcg
Chromium			50 mcg
N-acetyl cysteine	Proprietary amount	Proprietary amount	Proprietary amount
Coenzyme Q10	Proprietary amount	Proprietary amount	Proprietary amount
Alpha-lipoic acid	Proprietary amount	Proprietary amount	Proprietary amount
L-Carnitine	Proprietary amount		
Natural carotinoids	Proprietary amount	Proprietary amount	Proprietary amount
Resveratrol	Proprietary amount	Proprietary amount	Proprietary amount
Curcumin	Proprietary amount	Proprietary amount	Proprietary amount
Omega-3 fatty acids	Proprietary amount	Proprietary amount	Proprietary amount

Vitamin E
subcategories: supports mitochondirial health
Vitamin E functions as an antioxidant, reducing free radicals in the brain that would otherwise impede neuron function. Vitamin E has shown positive effects on memory performance in older people. An animal study showed a correlation between the amount of vitamin E ingested and improved neurologic performance, survival, and brain mitochondrial function.
Dietary Sources: Oils, nuts, spinach

Vitamin C
As a potent antioxidant, Vitamin C (ascorbic acid) appears to be particularly important in limiting lipid damage from free radicals. Studies have shown low levels of Vitamin C after a brain injury. It has been shown to help increase blood flow to the brain, and reduce injury size, neurological deficit, and mortality
Dietary Sources: Citrus fruits (such as oranges and grapefruit) and their juices, red and green pepper, kiwi, broccoli, strawberries, cantaloupe, baked potatoes, tomatoes

Vitamin D:
subcategories: seritonin enhancement
Many adolescents, adults, and elderly individuals are vitamin D deficient. In addition to being important in brain development, vitamin D provides important support to immune function, lowers the risk of autoimmune disorders, lowers the risk of cancer, and is important in maintaining normal mood

Dietary Sources: Cod liver oil, swordfish, salmon, tuna, orange juice (fortified), millk (fortified), yogurt (fortified), sardines, liver, egg, swiss cheese

Thiamine (Vitamin B1)
subcategories: supports mitochondirial health
Thiamine supports mitochondrial function in the brain by aiding the production of ATP. Thiamine is also an important co-factor, along with vitamin B12, in helping brain cells make myelin to insulate the nerve. As it is excreted by the kidneys, and generally not stored in the body, it is important to have a steady supply in one's diet
Dietary Sources: Tuna, Sunflower Seeds, Black Beans, Peas, Pinto Beans, Lentils, Lima Beans, Sesame Seeds

Riboflavin (Vitamin B2)
subcategories: supports mitochondirial health
Riboflavin is part of the complex of enzymes used by mitochondria to convert the energy stored in food to the energy stored in ATP to be used by the body. It is also a critical nutrient for the elimination of toxins
Dietary Sources: Almonds, fish, broccoli, asparagus. Most foods derived from plants or animals contain at least small quantities of riboflavin

Niacinamide (Vitamin B3)
subcategories: supports mitochondrial health
Niacinamide is an important nutrient for brain health. It is a key nutrient for mitochondria. An ample supply of niacinamide makes the generation of ATP more efficient and reduces the level of free radicals
Dietary Sources: Wheat germ, mushrooms, organ meats, tuna, salmon

Pyridoxine (Vitamin B6)
subcategories: supports mitochondrial health
Vitamin B6 is involved in many aspects of neurological activity. It is very important in forming many neurotransmitters, including serotonin and GABA
Dietary Sources: Garlic, tuna, cauliflower, mustard greens, bananas, celery, cabbage, crimini mushrooms, asparagus, broccoli, kale, collard greens, brussel sprouts, cod, chard.

Folic Acid
subcategories: supports mitochondirial health
Folatic acid is essential for normal brain function. It helps prevent hyperhomocysteinemia, which is associated with increased risk of heart disease, Parkinson's, Alzheimer's and other forms of dementia
Dietary Sources: Green leafy vegetables, asparagus, citrus fruit juices, legumes, fortified cereals

Cobolamin (Vitamin B12)
subcategories: supports mitochondrial health
The body needs cobolamin to make hemoglobin for the blood, and is necessary, along with vitamin B6, for brain cells to effectively make myelin, the protective sheath around nerve cells

Biotin
Biotin is a cofactor in synthesis and oxidation of fatty acids. It is also essential in the

process of carboxylation.
Dietary Sources: liver, rolled oats, eggs, milk, bananas, yeast, cheese, salmon, avocado, raspberries

Pantothenic Acid
It has been shown that pantothenic acid may improve the level of neurotransmitters and amino acids, which depend on the enzymatic activities of the Krebs cycle and linked to oxidative stress
Dietary Sources: animal organs (liver and kidney), fish, shellfish, milk products, eggs, avocados, legumes, mushrooms, sweet potatoes

Zinc glycinate:
Some people have shown zinc deficiency following a brain injury. In these cases supplementation may have a neuroprotective action, likely by affecting redox signaling. Due to mixed results regarding zinc, one must be cautious about not supplementing if there is no deficiency as it may worsen symptoms
Dietary Sources: Shellfish, meat (beef, pork, lamb, bison), poultry, fish, legumes (chickpeas, lentils, black beans, kidney beans, etc,), pumpkin seeds, cashews, hemp seeds, milk, yogurt, cheese, eggs, oats, quinoa, brown rice, mushrooms, kale, peas, asparagus, beet greens

Selenium:
subcategories: supports mitochondirial health
Selenium is a co-factor for the enzyme glutathione peroxidase, which helps generate glutathione in the mitochondria and has been shown to be neuroprotective.
Dietary Sources: fish, mushrooms, tofu, free-range chicken, turkey, venison

Chromium
Chromium is an essential nutrient required for optimal insulin activity and normal carbohydrate and lipid metabolism. Supplementation has been shown to increase tissue levels in deficiency, attenuate brain infarction, improve hyperglycemia, and decrease plasma levels of glucagon and corticosterone following brain injury
Dietary Sources: broccoli, liver, brewer's yeast, potatoes, whole grains, seafood, and meats

N-Acetyl Cysteine (NAC):
subcategories: glutathione enhancement
Considered the most cost-effective strategies to increase intracelluar glutathione, it is a key component in the generation of GABA. NAC has been shown to provide neuroprotection by reducing brain edema, blood-brain barrier permeability, and neuronal loss
Dietary Sources: poultry, yogurt, egg yolks, red peppers, garlic, onions, broccoli, brussel sprouts, other cruciferous vegetables, oats, wheat germ, asparagus, avocado

Co-enzyme Q
subcategories: supports mitochondirial health
Co-enzyme Q is an important ingredient in the mitochondrial process to generate ATP and it is a potent intracellular antioxidant.
Dietary Sources: wheat germ, dark green leafy vegetables like kale & spinach, organ meats

Alpha-Lipoic Acid

Several studies suggest that the use of alpha-lipoic acid may help reduce pain, burning, itching, tingling, and numbness in people who have nerve damage caused by diabetes. It has been shown to reduce inflammatory markers and oxidative stress while improving neuronal survival, preserving blood-brain-barrier permeability, and reducing edema.
Dietary Sources: Spinach, broccoli, beef, yeast (esp. brewer's yeast), kidney and heart organ meats

Acetyl- L-Carnitine
L-Carnitine is structurally related to the B vitamins and assists mitochondria in using fatty acids as an energy source. It also helps improve muscle strength in neuromuscular disorder affected individuals and has been associated with decreased oxidative stress and decreased aging in animal studies. L-Carnitine and Alpha Lipoic Acid have been shown to be a potent combination, providing protection to mitochondria and reducing aging in animals.
Dietary Sources: beef, pork, (meats raw or nearly raw for better absorption), poultry, fish, dairy products, cheese, avocado, asparagus

Natural Carotinoids
Lutein is one of the most prevalent carotinoids and most dominant throughout human brain tissue including areas controlling various aspects of cognition. It has neuroprotective and antioxidant properties and may influence interneuronal communication
Dietary Sources: yams, kale, spinach, watermelon, cantaloupe, bell peppers, carrots, mangoes, oranges

Resveratrol
Resveratrol has been the focus of a number of studies demonstrating it's antioxidant, anti-inflammatory, antimutagenic, and anticarcinogenic effects. [77-79] It has been shown that when administered immediately after a TBI it reduced oxidative damage and neuronal loss in rats. Recently it has been found resveratrol can mimic dietary restriction
Dietary Sources: Grapes, red wine, berries

Curcumin
There is substantial evidence that curcumin has anti-oxidant, anti-inflammatory, and antiamyloid activities. Studies have demonstrated that curcumin could cross the blood-brain barrier, targeting amyloid plaque buildups and disrupting existing plaques. [73]
Dietary Sources: Curry, used as a spice

Omega-3 Fatty Acids
Fish-derived omega-3 fatty acids have been shown to counteract deterioration in cognition and synaptic plasticity after traumatic brain injury. Docosahexaenoic acid (DHA) has been found to be a key component of neuronal membranes at neuron synapses. Evidence suggests DHA serves to improve neuronal function by supporting synaptic membrane fluidity and function, regulating gene expression and cell signaling. Omega-3 fatty acids also appear to reduce oxidative stress damage that results from trauma, indicating their possibility in facilitating the recovery process.
Dietary Sources: mackerel, salmon, cod liver oil, herrings, oysters, anchovies, sardines, caviar, flax seed, chia seeds, walnuts, soybeans

Other Dietary and Supplement Considerations

Magnesium:

subcategories: GABA enhancement/glutamate lowering

Magnesium blocks excessive stimulation from glutamate and decrease excito-toxicity when there is too much glutamate in the brain (often seen in those with MS, chronic pain, anxiety, seizures, and/or mood disorders). It has also been shown to be neuroprotective in animal models of brain injury.

Dietary Sources: Pumpkin seeds, sesame seeds, spinach, Swiss chard, black beans, pinto beans, milk of magnesia, epson salt baths

Organic Sulfur:

subcategories: GABA enhancement/glutamate lowering

A necessary component to generate the neurotransmitter GABA

Dietary Sources: Garlic, leeks, onion, chives, cabbage, kale, collards, broccoli, cauliflower, radishes, kohlrabi

Taurine:

subcategories: GABA enhancement/glutamate lowering

Taurine has been shown to help prevent epileptic seizures and be useful in the prevention of cardiac arrhythmias, atherosclerosis, and congestive heart failure. It has been suggested that 1-2 grams a day in divided doses may help GABA production in a strategy to protect the brain or assist in the treatment of mood disorders.

Dietary Sources: Fish, shellfish dark meat of turkey and chicken, milk, ice cream

Glutathione:

Very important to the generation of GABA. It is manufactured inside the cell, from 'its precursor amino acids: glycine, glutamate and cysteine.

Dietary Sources: Must be manufactured from it's precursors, particularly cysteine.

Dietary Polyphenols

Polyphenols can be broadly divided into two categories: flavonoids and non-flavonoids. Although numerous studies have reported flavonoid-mediated neuroprotection, there is little information about the interaction of flavonoids or their metabolites with the blood-brain barrier. The flavonoid epigallocatechin gallate has been reported to enter the brain after gastric administration. The citrus flavonoids naringin and hesperetin readily cross the blood-brain barrier, whereas glucuronide or glycoside conjugates do not do so as easily.

Theanine:

Shown to be neuroprotective as well as improving cognition and concentration and reducing anxiety and depression

Dietary Sources: Green tea – particularly matcha tea

Citicoline

An acetylcholine precursor that readily crosses the blood-brain-barrier, citicoline has been shown in animal studies to prevent TBI-induced neuronal loss in the hippocampus, decrease brain lesion size, and improve neurologic recovery. It additionally improved mitochondrial lipid metabolism and phospholipid synthesis. In humans, studies have shown increased cerebral blood flow, decreased infarct volume, accelerated recovery of consciousness, and improved recovery of cognitive, memory, verbal, and motor deficits.

SAMe

SAMe maintains cellular membrane integrity in repairing damaged proteins and maintaining lipid fluidity in nerve cell membranes. It also generates glutathione, the body's major antioxidant, and enhances the function of the dopamine system.

Creatine Monohydrate
subcategories: supports mitochondrial health
Creatine functions to increase the availability of ATP. Several studies have shown that taking additional creatine has been neuroprotective to a variety of injuries and has helped maintain and improve muscle strength in people with Parkinson's and the frail elderly. *Dietary Sources:* Fish, red meat, wild game, organ meats

Fasting and the Ketogenic Diet
Fasting has been studied in rat models of brain injury with results showing that fasting for 24 hours, but not 48 hours, after a moderate, but not severe, injury showed neuroprotection with significant tissue sparing, preservation of cognitive functioning, and improvement of mitochondrial function. Biomarkers for oxidative stress were also shown to be decreased.

Ketone administration after a moderate injury also showed tissue sparing.[4] TBI patients who were fasted or maintained on a ketogenic-like diet to minimize hyperglycemia have also demonstrated significantly lower plasma glucose and lactate concentrations, elevated β-hydroxybutyrate levels, and better urinary nitrogen balance compared to a normal diet.

Because of this it has been argued that whether ketosis is achieved by starvation or administration of a ketogenic diet, the common underlying conditions of low plasma glucose in the presence of ketones have consistently shown neuroprotective effects after a brain injury and that maintenance of "normoglycemia" may not be the optimal approach post-injury. A combination of ketone administration and saline has also been shown to potentially provide added control of intracranial pressure with improved cerebral metabolism. [4] Little exploration into specific dosing, timing and route/duration of administration has been done however, so caution should be taking a ketogenic approach as side effects including dehydration, hypoglycemia, and (less commonly) nutrient deficiency, decreased bone density, immune dysfunction, cardiomyopathy, and elevated blood cholesterol with a prolonged ketogenic diet.[6]

Positive Affirmations
Maintaining a positive attitude during the recovery process can be very helpful for one's mental state as well as actually helping the healing process forward and working to keep motivated. Some helpful affirmations may include:
-"No matter what my symptoms, my health is improving every second"
-"I am thankful for the healing that is restoring my body"
-"I am willing to accept what happened and I choose to overcome"
-"My body will follow my ,mind, and my mid will demand full recovery"
-"I am more than my injuries. I am more than my pain. I am a healing force"
-"Miracles come to those who believe, and I believe"
-"If I can visualize it, I can achieve it, and I can see myself become whole again

Charting and keeping record of progress and achievements in the healing process can be very helpful in being able to look back at how far someone has come over time, even if some days feel like none has been made or seems too hard.

Chapter 7
Plants and Herbs – Phytotherapeutics

There are a number of plant and mineral based substances that have been shown to have benefit and pharmacological effects following a brain injury or aiding in the recovery process. Due to the majority of my training being rooted in Chinese medicine, some of the substances may be better known within the Chinese medicine pharmacopoeia and I have included their Chinese names in parentheses.

Berries
Berries are a rich source of phenolic compounds as well as anthocyanins and other flavenoids which have shown significant antioxidant effect. In mice supplemented with blueberry extract, hippocampal concentrations of proteins involved in early and late stages of memory formation. [71] This indicate that blueberry extract supplementation might prevent cognitive and motor deficits through various neuronal signaling pathways.

Green Tea
Green tea is rich in flavonoids, including catechin which has been associated with a wide variety of health benefits. The prevention of stroke has been demonstrated, and several studies have shown that green tea extract may protect neurons from A-beta-induced damage as found in Alzheimer's disease .[75-77] It has been shown to minimize oxidative damage and reduce neuronal cell death.[78]

Huperzine A
An extract of Chinese club moss, this is a potent selective reversible acetylcholinesterase inhibitor. Being rapidly absorbed and easily crossing the blood-brain barrier, it has demonstrated positive outcomes in vascular dementia and cognitive decline.

Pine Needle
Pre-treatment with pine needle extract has shown to protect hippocampal neurogenesis suppressed by scopolamine by facilitating BDNF and modulating cholinergic activity.[1] Another study showed pine needle polyphenols significantly increased antioxidative capacity, glutathione, and super oxide dismutase activity, while nitric oxide activity was decreased, showing a significant relieving effect on learning, memory, and spontaneous activities.[2]

Milk Thistle
subcategories: Glutathione enhancement
A powerful antioxidant that supports the brain, liver and kidneys by preventing the depletion of glutathione. Silymarin is the active compound in milk thistle and is considered helpful in the detoxification process of the liver as well as protecting the liver from toxins.
Dietary Sources: Milk thistle seeds

Ginkgo Biloba (Yin Xing Ye)
Ginkgo has been shown to increase blood flow to the brain while crossing the blood-brain-barrier and aiding in memory. Compounds within Gingko have shown potent free radical scavenging and antioxidant effects that likely play a role in its neuroprotective properties. Enhancement of the cholinergic system in various brain regions have been shown with

increases in acetyl-choline release in hippocampal neurons. Benefits have been shown in behavioral measures of spatial working memory and increasing the density of hippocampal muscarinic receptors.

Turmeric (Yu Jin)
subcategories: Glutathione enhancement
A powerful anti-oxidant , anti-inflammatory, and anti-amyloid substance. Turmeric is believed to inhibit lipid peroxidation, activate glutathione, or induce heme oxygenase. Studies have demonstrated that turmeric could cross the blood-brain barrier, targeting amyloid plaques and disrupting existing plaques. It has been shown to effectively lower oxidative damage, cognitive deficits, synaptic marker loss, and amyloid deposition while inhibiting cytokine and microglial activation related to neurotoxicity
*Dietary Sources:*Curry, used as a spice

Red Sage Root (Dan Shen)
The benefits of salvia in promoting circulation, particularly capillary microcirculation, and alleviating fibrosis have been extensively researched[7]. Neuroprotective effects have been shown from the herb, especially in relation to Parkinson's disease and stroke. In a stroke model where the blood-brain-barrier was penetrated, brain infarct volume was reduced by 30% and 37% following treatment with it's two primary active constituents. This was accompanied by a significant decrease in neurological deficit.[11] It has also been shown in protecting diverse cells from damage caused by a variety of toxic stimuli, likely due to its antioxidative and anti-apoptotic activity.

Scutellaria (Huang Qin)
The flavonoids of scutellaria have been studied extensively because they show a potent and broad therapeutic benefit with no signs of toxicity in moderately high clinical doses. Key components have been isolated and evaluated for anti-inflammatory and neuroprotective actions. Wogonin is a potent neuroprotector that has shown inhibition of inflammatory activation of microglia. In animal models wogonin showed neuroprotection by reducing death of hippocampal neurons by reducing microglia inflammation. [8] It has also been shown to reduce total injury site size in the cerebral cortex and striatum while significantly improving behavioral deficits. Scutellaria has also been shown to ameliorate blood-brain barrier permeability in breaches due to injury.

Panax Ginseng (Ren Shen)
Ginseng is one of the most widely used of all traditional Chinese herbs. Its neuroprotective effects have been shown in increased neurite outgrowth in the absence of nerve growth factor (NGF) suggesting neurotrophic actions that may contribute to reported enhancement of cognitive function. [13] Nitric oxide and cytokines, which have been implicated in chronic brain inflammation, have been shown to be significantly inhibited. Ginseng acts on hormonal, immune, and metabolic functions while enhancing general physical and mental health. In terms of influence on intelligence, ginsenosides promote reflexes, reactions, memory, and thinking processes. Through MAO inhibition it is beneficial in the synthesis of neural transmitters, thus enhancing overall brain function.

Acorus (Shi Chang Pu)
Acorus has been demonstrated as a potent free radical scavenger which can lower excitatory amino acids and have a protective effect on the brain by decreasing levels of aspartic acid

and taurine levels in brain tissue.[1] Chronic use of acorus has shown an increase in alpha activity, along with an increase in norepinephrine levels in the cerebral cortex but a decrease in the midbrain and cerebellum. Serotonin levels were raised in the cerebral cortex but decreased in the midbrain. Similarly, dopamine level was increased in the caudate nucleus and midbrain but decreased in the cerebellum. From this it was concluded acorus seems to exert its depressive action by changing electrical activity and brain monoamine levels in different brain regions.[4] It's classical indication to "open the mind" has been verified by it's ability to increase permeability of the blood-brain barrier. [5] This quality makes it particularly useful in cases of brain injury to direct other herbal medicines to the brain and allow for increased cerebral blood flow.

Acanthopanax (*Ci Wu Jia*)
Animal studies have shown the strong anti-inflammatory and pain relieving effects of Acanthopanax[10] along with its effects in the prevention of multiple organ dysfunction.[11] It is also known to have healing and protective effects on stress-induced mental disturbances. Animal studies have suggested that Acanthopanax may act by regulating noradrenaline (NA) and dopamine (DA) levels in specific brain regions related to the stress response.[12]

Schizandra (Wu Wei Zi)
Schizandra excites the central nervous system, increases brain efficiency, and regulates the cardiovascular system to improve circulation. It has shown some effect in enhancing impaired intelligence/cognition.

Ligusticum (Chuan Xiong)
Used to promote Blood circulation to remove stasis. Ligusticum has been proven to significantly increase cerebral blood flow and inhibit abnormalities such as slow blood flow, granular and cottonlike blood flow patterns, RBC aggregation, microembolus and degeneration and necrosis of nerve tissue.

Astragalus (Huang Qi)
Astragalus is a tonifying herb which aids blood flow as a cardiotonic and vasodilator, reduces hypotensive symptoms, has antibacterial actions, boosts the immune system, slows the aging process (by lengthening telomeres), and has an adaptogen-like regulating effect. It's intellectual functions may be attributed to it's ability to inhibit MAO, thus increasing the transmitters that influence excitation of the brain and cerebral blood flow.

Polygonum (He Shou Wu/Shou Wu Teng)
Polygonum is an outstanding herb for slowing the aging process. It has been demonstrated in lowering cholesterol, preventing atherosclerosis, and action as a cardiotonic. In the central nervous system, it has a stimulatory action and inhibits monoamine oxidase (MAO).

Gastrodia (Tian Ma)
Gastrodia is widely used by TCM physicians to manage headache, dizziness, vertigo, dementia, and convulsions [37]. Pharmacological studies have shown that the anticonvulsive properties and brain neuronal protective effects of the constituents of Gastrodia are related to their free radical scavenging activities and modulator effects on neurotransmission [36, 38-41]. The cognitive benefits of Gastrodia and its ability to improve learning and memory have been confirmed by animal studies. [42-44]

Polygala (Yuan Zhi)

Polygala is an herb primarily indicated in helping to "calm the mind", assisting in symptoms such as insomnia, anxiety, restlessness. It has been shown to have cytoprotective properties against neurotoxicity while increasing nerve growth factor (NGF) and brain-derived neurotrophic factor (BDNF). Polygala also has a demonstrated rapid onset anti-depressive effect by modulating glutametergic synapses in the hippocampus and other critical brain circuits.

Essential Oils

Essential oil qualities can vary greatly: antibacterial, anti-inflammatory, immunostimulant with hormonal, glandular, emotional, circulatory, and calming effects, as well as memory and alertness enhancement have been documented.[8, 9] The stimulation properties of these oils are said to lay in their structure that closely resemble with actual hormones.[10] The mechanism of action is said to involve integration of oils into a biological signal of the receptor cells in the nose when inhaled. The signal is then transmitted to limbic and hypothalamic regions of the brain via olfactory bulb.

These signals cause the brain to release neurotransmitters like serotonin, norepinephrine, etc. to link the nervous system and other body systems to elicit a healing response.[11] The olfactory bulb has been shown to continue neurogenesis into adulthood.[12] This, coupled with the connections to the limbic system and hippocampus, may point to particular scents and stimulation of the bulb potentially changing cognitive patterns of memories or traumas. The matter of essential oils is a common question given it's rise in popularity in recent years. As such, I have included some oils which may be given consideration based on possible evidence.

Bergamot
A study demonstrated bergamot essential oil to reduce neuronal damage caused in vitro by excitotoxic stimuli and that the neuroprotection prevented neuronal death, reactive oxygen species accumulation, and activation of calpain. This is was hypothesized to be the result of oil monoterpene hydrocarbons.[8]

Basil
Basil is a top note oil which is listed as a nervine, CNS stimulant and adrenal restorative. It is indicated for concussion, fatigue, exhaustion, nervous depression, anxiety, memory loss, and shock.

Frankincense/Boswellia
Frankincense is a base note oil that, among other things, is said to act as a nervous restorative, antidepressant, antioxidant and immunostimulant. In herbal form frankincense is known as Ru Xiang and used in Chinese medicine frequently for it's anti-inflammatory, analgesic, and wound healing properties indicated for traumas of many types. As an oil some of it's indications include irritability, restlessness, sensory overstimulation, nightmares, mental confusion or weakness, neurasthenia and menstrual irregularities.

Vetiver
Vetiver is a base note oil well regarded as having a relaxant or grounding effect in overstimulation conditions. It is listed as being indicated for anxiety, fear, hypersensitivity,

overexcitment, delusion, and paranoia. It is also said to reduce hyperactive basal ganglia and cingulate systems and resolve temporal lobe dysregulation. It is said to be a neuroendocrine restorative, assisting in hormonal or central nervous system deficiencies including fatigue, chronic neurasthenia, insomnia, and hysteria. A study of it's chemical constituents concluded vetiver oil may suppress inflammatory responses including nitric oxide production and cell apoptosis.[9]

Lavender
A top/middle note, lavender oil has been studied and shown to have growing evidence of offering benefit in several neurological disorders. Several animal and human studies suggest anxiolytic, mood stabilizer, sedative, analgesic, and anticonvulsive and neuroprotective properties. Rat studies have shown to diminish glutamate-induced neurotoxicity[11] as well as decreasing neurological deficit scores, infarct size, and the levels of mitochondria-generated reactive oxygen species, and neuronal damage.[12]

Orange
Orange essential oil, a top note, has been found to have CNS depressant-like effects in mice. A study examined the effects on fear memory and immune cell activation in a mouse model of PTSD using Pavlovian Fear Conditioning. This study suggests that orange oil may affect extinction of fear memories.[13]

Chapter 8
Body-Based Approaches

Functional Neurology
Functional neurology is a an approach by a natural healthcare provider who has done additional post-doctoral training in neurological testing and treatment protocols. Based on assessment, a wide range of "receptor-based" treatment approaches may be used. Part of the foundation of functional neurology lies in the central integrative state (CIS) of neurons and neural groups. This is the total received input by a neuron and it's probability of creating an action potential based on it's level of functionability along with the rate and length of time the nervous system takes to respond. Based on this and other assessments precise exercises and methods of sensory input are used to stimulate parts of the nervous system to improve their function.

Treatment goals are generally composed of the following strategies
-Modulating the central integrative state of the system to maximize neuron function
-Promote regeneration of neurons while decreasing neuron loss
-Stimulate a repair process in any injured neurons
-Promote neuroplasticity
-Assist oxygen delivery to the system
-Ensure adequate fuel and other necessary

Beyond standard neurological testing they may use additional visual, vestibular, and balance testing to determine what approaches are best suited for the individual.
This may include
-vestibular therapy
-vision therapy
-physical exercises
-gait retraining
-laser, vibration, and/or electrical stimulation
-neurosensory integration therapy
as well as other modalities explored in the rest of this chapter

Biofeedback and Neurofeedback
Biofeedback is an umbrella term for a number of treatments that use conditioning to help people become more aware of their own bodily responses in real time and, with practice and feedback, learn to control these once-automatic responses better in order to reduce symptoms, improve performance, and/or increase well-being. A variety of factors including surface temperature, heart rate variability, muscle tension, skin conductance, and EEG are used, either singly or together, to transmit the data to the user, usually via visual and/or audio displays, while the user is guided by a trained clinician. Reinforcements like controlling elements of a computer game based on body changes help train users to become more aware of and ultimately control their responses to emotional, cognitive, or physical stimuli. Users can then learn to alter the behaviors, habits, patterns, and responses that are contributing to symptoms or affecting performance or function.

People with headaches or attention problems following a brain injury for example may have a protocol involving a general stress and relaxation assessment, using multiple types of biofeedback to measure their response to stressors—such as solving math problems out loud, or recalling an emotionally stressful event, or having to pay close attention to a detail-oriented task—as well as their ability to relax following the stressor. Approaches would then be used to alter the body in ways that reduce symptoms and/or improve performance.

Biofeedback in general for symptoms related to TBI often varies depending on the type, severity, symptomatology, and duration of the brain injury. There are varied protocols and approaches to using the many types of biofeedback, many of which are used in combination with more than one form of biofeedback at the same time, and are also often used in conjunction with other forms of therapy, such as cognitive behavioral therapy.

Neurofeedback
The use of EEG biofeedback (neurofeedback), while not the only type of biofeedback used for brain injury, has become a common and promising choice for the treatment of TBI by measuring outputs and patterns of the affected organ and comparing them to associated cognitive states and processes.

EEG patterns have been shown to be different in individuals following TBI, and have even been shown to predict prognosis in some cases. Side-effects from neurofeedback can include headaches, nausea, dizziness, fatigue, and agitation. These are common symptoms that TBI survivors seek to mitigate that might be worsened by the use of a computer screen used to provide feedback.

As with other forms of biofeedback, the principles of helping train users to become more of aware of the patterns that might be contributing to symptoms and/or interfering with performance, and learning to change these patterns through real-time audio, visual, and/or sensory feedback, is the same. The number of sessions required in order to achieve positive change may range from 5 to 60, sometimes involving more than 1 session per week to help generalize skills and improve outcomes. One may be guided to help increase attention or concentration, or helped to decrease activity in certain areas by using relaxation techniques, for example, which are thought to contribute to neural plasticity.

Neurofeedback research has documented its value in the treatment of a variety of symptoms relevant to a brain injury population, including seizures, memory, concentration and attention, unstable mood, impulsiveness, anxiety, depression, sleep issues, and even anosmia and physical balance. Research for veteran populations has often focused on its use when PTSD or substance abuse also exist alongside TBI from blast injuries, and have shown significant improvements.

Massage
Various styles of massage can be helpful to alleviate muscle tension and pain. Headaches can be alleviated by reducing tension in the neck or scalp areas. Acupressure can be applied to points indicated for specific functions. Positional release techniques, a form of passive movement aimed at alleviating muscle and tendon tension such as the Japanese technique Sotai can be helpful in cases of contracture and mobility limitations. The sensory stimulation of bodywork sends neural signals to the sensory-motor cortex in the parietal lobe. This creates a feedback promoting peripheral nerve regeneration and reduction in inflammation.

CranioSacral therapy

One specific approach which may be particularly helpful following a brain injury is craniosacral therapy. Anatomically, the craniosacral system is the deepest layer of the connective tissue (fascia) system, a continuous network surrounding every structure of the body. It's structure is relatively simple. The cranium is lined with dura mater, which not only encircles the inner surfaces of the cranial bones, but also folds in on itself creating what's known as the intracranial membrane. This continues downward with attachments to the upper cervical vertebra of the neck (C1 and C2). It then continues further downward without any attachments until it anchors at the lower spine a little above the tailbone (S2 of the sacrum). It exits out of the sacral canal and ends at the tailbone. The dura mater also extends out through the holes in the spinal vertebra (foramina) with the spinal nerves known as dural sleeves that blend into the rest of the body's connective tissue.

The premise of craniosacral is that restricted cranial bone movement reflects not only restrictions of the suture between the bones, but of underlying meninges attaching to the bone. CST techniques address both types of limitations in movement. A concussion affects the structures of the nervous system including the glial cells. This glial matrix, while different from fascia, shares some similar functions by transporting nutritive substances and removing waste products through the extracellular matrix. Disturbances of this fluid may impact communication between brain regions.

It is suspected that the positive results experienced with craniosacral therapy in post concussion syndrome results by affecting not only the dura and cranial bones but also the glial network attaching directly to brain structures they support. Techniques include mobilization of each of the bones around its anatomical axis affecting the attaching membrane and the glial network that attaches directly to the meninges of the nervous system. Examples include a "frontal lift technique" which can address tension patterns related to the frontal lobe. This can affect behavioral changes associated with impaired decision making and focus. Temporal techniques may address tinnitus and dizziness symptoms. Post Concussion Syndrome and associated symptoms have been shown to clinically responded to craniosacral.

Hyperbaric Oxygen Therapy

Hyperbaric Oxygen Therapy, abbreviated HBO or HBOT, is a medical treatment that uses high dose oxygen to speed and enhance the body's natural ability to heal. HBOT is approved by the American Medical Association, FDA, and Medicare. Persons who may benefit from HBOT suffer from various diseases or injuries associated with a lack of oxygen at the cellular level (hypoxia) and aids in boosting mitochondrial metabolism.

Oxygen is dissolved into all of the body's fluids, plasma, the central nervous system fluids, the lymph, and the bone, carrying it to areas where circulation has been diminished or blocked. The increased oxygen concentration can enhance the ability of white blood cells to kill bacteria, reduce swelling, and allow new blood vessels to grow more rapidly into the affected areas.

In many cases, such as circulatory problems, non-healing wounds, and strokes, adequate oxygen cannot reach the damaged area and the body's natural healing ability is unable to function properly.

-Increases tissue oxygenation in the brain
-Slows and reverses hypoxic induced apoptosis
-Restores blood supply to the compromised region of the brain
-Generates new capillary networks (neovascularization)
-Aids other regenerative therapies, such as PRP and stem cell therapies

Studies show the effectiveness of hyperbaric oxygen treatment in improving brain function and quality of life in mild traumatic brain injury (mTBI) patients suffering chronic neurocognitive impairments. The common conclusion is that HBOT can induce neuroplasticity, leading to repair of chronically impaired brain functions and improved quality of life in those with TBI or prolonged post-concussion syndrome (PCS) at late chronic stage. Studies also show that HBOT can reduce cognitive impairment related to memory performance and connectivity using functional MRI.

Hyperbaric oxygen treatment has been shown to decrease swelling, repair the metabolic injury to the neuron cells, and stop the inflammation in acute brain injuries with just a few treatments in the first 72 hours after injury. It is the only intervention currently known to break the cycle, after which neurological function can be worked to be restored.

Manual Manipulations (Adjustments)

Vertebral joint manipulations have been reported to have an effect on numeous signs and symptoms related to central nervous system function including visual dysfunction, reaction time, central motor excitability, dizziness, tinnitus or hearing impairment, migraine, jaw clenching, bipolar and sleep disturbances, and neck dystonia.

A number of potential pathways exist that may explain why spinal and joint manipulations have the potential to have modulatory effects on the brain through exitement of the rostral ventrolateral medulla. These include:

-Cervical manipulations excite spinoreticular paythwyas and spinocerebellar pathways

-Cervical manipulations modulate the vestibulosympathetic pathways

-Cervical manipulations cause vestibulocerebellar activation of regions of the vagus nerve

-May result in brain hemisphere influences causing descending excitation of the pontomedullary reticular formation (PMRF)

-Lumbosacral manipulations may result in sympathetic modulation

-Spinal manipulations may alter the expression of segmental somatosympatethic reflexes by reducing small fiber afferent imput and enhancing large fiber afferent input

-Spinal manipulations may alter the expression of suprasegmental somatosympathetic reflexes by reducing afferent inputs on second-order ascending spinoreticular neurons which may influence the immune system on a global level

88

-Spinal manipulations may alter central integration of brainstem cneters involved in somatosympathetic relfexes

-Spinal manipulations may alter central integration in the hypothalamus and the influence of spinal afferents on vestibular and midline cerebellar functions.

-Spinal manipulations may influence brain asymmetry by enhancing neurons in the central nervous system or brainstem, or cerebral blood flow through autonomic influences

Acupuncture and Chinese Medicine

A significant advantage to the use of Chinese medical and natural treatment approaches is their relative safety and low risk of negative ("side") effects. With acupuncture, the primary risks are minimal and infrequent: mild bruising, numbness and tingling may occur at the insertion sight, hematomas are rare but may also occur. An individual may begin to feel dizzy or light headed during or for a short duration immediately following a treatment. If performed improperly there is a risk of puncturing of the lung or other organs, nerve damage or infection due to non-sterile conditions. So long as the practitioner has done adequate and proper training, the likelihood of these occurring are minuscule. For the patient seeking treatment however, this is an important reason to make sure their provider has completed adequate training in a full Chinese medical curriculum.

Chinese herbal medicine can often be used to address many symptoms related to brain injury as well as help facilitate the overall healing process. Many individual herbs are listed withing this text. Herbal combinations and specific remedies can be found in my previous book *"Healing Brain Injury with Chinese Medical Approaches"*.

Acupuncture Mechanisms

Local Effects – Pain reduction, anti-inflammatory effects, initiation of the healing response
The insertion of an acupuncture needle into the skin, in essence, creates a type of microinjury. While this is not enough to cause actual damage to the area, it is a breaching of the epidermis, which alerts the body to respond in a number of various ways. Upon needle insertion, an "axon reflex" occurs throughout the meshwork of surrounding nerves. This stimulates local muscle fibers. Through this there is a triggering of a powerful vasodilator (CGRP), which opens local capillaries and releases various neuropeptides from local mast cells. This release downregulates the pain cascade, works to reduce inflammation in the area, initiates the healing response of tissue, fights infections and increases local circulation. The local tissue cells can also stimulate vascular nerve fibers which triggers nitric oxide (NO) production. Other tissues that may be involved include smooth muscle cells and endothelium cells as a result of NO production which further increases the blood flow and local circulation.[5]

Acupuncture is thought to have it's pain killing effect through the release of local endorphins, the body's natural opioids, and of the neurotransmitter encephalin, which inhibits the pain pathway as a means of " hyperstimulation". Studies have also shown acupuncture to effectively trigger an increase in ATP[6,] a key component in energy exchange during metabolic processes, around the insertion site. By increasing ATP the body is better able to create both a well-recognized pain-reducing effect, but also contribute more usable energy and innate healing potential within the body.

Acupuncture regulates homeostatic states (somatic autonomic reflex) of both the sympathetic and parasympathetic branches of the autonomic nervous system to reinstate a balanced dynamic between the two.When an acupuncture needle is inserted into the desired acupoint, there are several different peripheral afferent fibers that can be found in the area of insertion. These have been shown to be in greater abundance at acupuncture points compared to non-points along the body. Surface oxygen levels have also been shown to be in higher concentrations at locations of traditional acupuncture points.[7]

Effects on Muscles
Areas within the muscle where the nerve stimulates movement can be used to treat pain in the area, loosen a tight muscles, or to improve range of motion or mobility. These are often known as muscle motor points, trigger points, or traditionally "ashi" points. Here the primary incoming pain-relief system which connects to the emotional regions of the brain become stimulated. This may help to "reset" the muscle to a state of relaxation. Gunn[8] uses the term intramuscular stimulation rather than acupuncture when referring to the needling process for this reason. In this sense it has been argued that acupuncture may be considered a variation of cortisone injection within myofascial trigger points. In the case of neuralgias and neuropathies acupuncture stimulation may have a local effect on restoring the diseased nerve by improving the local blood flow and accelerating cellular metabolism.

Spinal Segmental Effects – Acupuncture Analgesia and the "Gate Theory"
All pain-reducing fibers enter the spinal column, it is here that neurotransmitters, including serotonin and norepinephrine are released which lessens pain signals. This also relaxes the smooth muscle of the nerve segment, which then releases unnecessary stress on the organ, increases circulation, and aids in enhancing the organ's function. This accounts for effects of "distal acupuncture" where points are inserted in areas of the body other than where the trouble area is.

Fascia Structure Effects
It has been shown by various researchers that the fascia (connective tissue) planes throughout the body form a network that resembles the meridians traditionally described in Chinese medicine.[9,10,11]

The nerves within these fascial planes carry signals throughout. In essence, when the acupuncture needle is inserted into the connective tissue, the fascia responds and "wraps" around the needle in response. This results in a mechanical force within muscle tissue which propagates to neighboring muscles. This signal creates a rippling response downstream resulting in changes in fascia or anti-inflammatory response. Other signals such as paracrine-signaling molecules[12] and piezoelectric signals throughout the liquid crystalline structure[13,14] of the fascial network have also been shown.

Endogenous Opioid Circuit (EOC) Effects
The hypothalamus is one of the largest manufacturers of beta-endorphins, our naturally produced opioids, which reduce pain. Signals from acupuncture insertion make their way to the hypothalamus and these opioids immediately bring down all pain signaling. Opioid release has been studied extensively in treatment of addiction disorders utilizing electro-acupuncture. Specific millicurrent frequencies have shown to elicit greater releases of particular endorphins.[15]

Central Nervous System and Disease Treatment Effects
Acupuncture effects the hormonal/endocrine systems by stimulating the hypothalamus which influences the anterior pituitary and ultimately the adrenals, having an impact on the entire network called the hypothalamic-pituitary axis (HPA). Regulation happens throughout the HPA through acupuncture stimulus arriving at the higher brain centers after passing through the limbic system. This induces the higher brain to initiate the needed commands which passes to the hypothalamus for final execution of endocrine, autonomic, and other homeostasic tasks.

Effects on the immune system take place through general autonomic changes in the lymphoreticular system of the marrow and spleen. Endorphins are released into the blood stream with demonstrated increases in natural killer cells and changes in gamma- interferon levels.

Acupuncture Activates and Deactivates different areas of the Brain
Results of functional magnetic resonance imaging (fMRI) studies have shown that stimulation at a traditional acupuncture point create responses in specific areas of the brain compared to needling non-acupuncture points. Studies have also demonstrated "point specificity" in which different points affect different areas of the brain.

A review of studies showed"acupuncture treatments were associated with more activation, mainly in the somatosensory areas, motor areas, basal ganglia, cerebellum, limbic system and higher cognitive areas (e.g. prefrontal cortex). Three studies also showed more deactivation in the limbic system in response to acupuncture."[18]

Acupuncture has also been shown to have the ability to increase glucose metabolism and improve cerebral blood flow in the brain areas related to cognition and memory by increasing glucose transporter 1 (GLUT1) which is involved in cellular respiration, regulation of glucose levels and vitamin C uptake. Studies Indicated that upregulation of GLUT1 by acupuncture alleviates cognitive impairment resulting from lack of blood and/or oxygen.[20]

Acupuncture Increases Neuroplasticity and Neurogenesis
Particularly relevant to the treatment of brain injuries is how acupuncture has been shown to have a direct influence on neuroplasticity (ability to form new connections) and neurogenesis (ability to create new neurons) within the brain. Until relatively recently it was thought that any neuronal loss due to injury or aging in adults could not be repaired. It is now known that neural stem cells are still active in certain regions of the adult brain (namely the dentate gyrus of the hippocampus and the subventricular zones). While this ability is now known to exist in adults, it is still much slower than in children.

A recent study showed that acupuncture induced cell and neuroblast differentiation in the hippocampus, providing evidence that it may be useful as a neurogenesis-stimulating therapy. It has also been shown to affect cAMP signaling, a transcription factor important in proliferation, differentiation, and survival of neural precursor cells. Regulation of neurotrophic factor which supports the growth, differentiation and survival of neurons has also been demonstrated. The following acupuncture points have been shown to influence neuronal proliferation:

ST-36   GV-20   PC-6

91

HT-7	SP-10	TW-5
CV-17	GV-16	GB-30
CV-12	GV-8	
CV-6	LI-11	

One of the most studied and clinically used points among these is ST-36, located on the lower leg. Simulation of ST-36 is used for a wide range of conditions affecting the digestive, cardiovascular system, immune and nervous systems, as well as having been widely used for brain disorders. In addition to this, ST-36 was shown to upregulate the expression of neuropeptide Y, which promotes proliferation of neuronal precursor cells and appeared to lessen nerve damage.[21]

Two points on the head, GV-20 and GV-26, regulated cells which "increase the release of nerve growth factors (NGF) to make nerve cells survive and axons grow, synthesize neurotransmitters, (and) metabolize toxic substances." Similarly the use of GV-20 and GV-14 was shown to increase neural repair after ischemic damage. These points also activate bodily self-protection and reduction of nerve cell death in and near the site of injury. Needling points along the midline of the torso, traditionally called the conception vessel, were shown to increase growth factors - basic fibroblast growth factor, epidermal growth factor and NGF messenger RNA - in the subventricular zones and dentate gyrus.[22]

Scalp Acupuncture
The majority of acupuncture points are located on the trunk and limbs. However, the points along the surface of the head play an important role in addressing sequelae of brain injury with acupuncture. GV-20, located at the top of the head, has been shown to increase cerebral blood flow velocity without significant changes in blood pressure and pulse rate.[23] Specific scalp acupuncture systems and protocols are a relatively new, yet promising, method to treating brain injury and its related symptoms[24-26]. Several scalp "systems" exist, including needling over the sensory-motor humunculi along the parietal and frontal lobes to increase both movement and sensory feedback..

Part 3

Common Symptoms

Chapter 9
Headache/Migraine

According to the International headache society, a post-traumatic headache is defined as one that starts within 7 days of the injury or returning to a conscious state following TBI. It may spontaneously resolve over the next 6 months or it may become chronic.

Post-traumatic headache is more prevalent in cases of mild TBI (95% of those reporting pain) compared to moderate-to-severe TBI (22% of those reporting pain). Nearly 1/3 of soldiers returning from deployment who sustained a concussion met criteria for post-traumatic headache. A recent study showed 40-50% of patients with TBI reporting headache at 3, 6, and 12 months. A chronic headache is defined as one which occurs at least 15 days per month for at least three months. This must also not be linked to any type of medication overuse or withdrawal.

Looking at the neurological structure of the head and neck, there are multiple receptors that may be affected. These receptors are located at the end of nerves that begin near the spinal cord and communicate with pain centers of the brain. The nerves carrying signals to the brain that could possibly involved in post-traumatic headache include:
Cranial Nerve V (trigeminal)
Cranial Nerve IX (glossopharyngeal)
Cranial Nerve X (vagus)
Greater Occipital Nerve (C2 root origin)
Lesser Occipital Nerve (C3 root origin)

It is important to for practitioners to distinguish if a headache is a primary symptom or if it may the secondary result of another medical problem.

Common Diagnostic Testing
-CBC (complete blood count)
-Chem screen
-ESR (erythrocyte sedimentation rate)
-Glucose
-Urinalysis
-CSF (cerebral spinal fluid collection)
-EENT
-X-ray
-MRI
-CT scan

Possible Confounding Factors

-Stress
-Muscle tension
-Eyestrain, visual defects
-Fevers, sinusitis
-Occupation
-Toxic/environmental exposure
-Allergies
-Improper yoga, exercise
-Family history

Headache Types

Non-vascular
Tension Headache

Tension headaches are the most common form of primary headache. Related to head trauma, rates at one year after injury were 38.3% for episodic and 2.2% for chronic tension headaches. Stemming from muscle spasm or postural sprain, tension headaches are estimated to make up 70% of all non-vascular headaches.

Qualities
-Gradual onset as muscle tension builds with cycles of tension and relaxation.
-Often affect both sides of head like a band of pressure around the head. Pain relatively mild
-Muscles of the neck and skull often tender to palpation.
-Muscle strain causes inflammation and noxious stimuli release (seritonin, bradykinin, histamine, and prostaglandins)
-Common pathways involved in many migraines
-Not associated with aura, nausea, vomiting, or sensitivity to light and sound.
-Physical activity does not tend to impact pain intensity.

Tension Headache Treatment Considerations
-NSAIDs and OTC pain medication– Aspirin, Ibuprofen (Motrin, Advil), Acetaminophen (Tylenol), Naproxen (Aleve)
-Antidepressants, anticonvulsants, Botox
-Acupuncture
-Massage, Physiotherapy
-Therabands and resistive exercise systems
-Biofeedback, stress management

Cervicogenic Headache

This refers to head pain that is generated from the cervical spine.
C1-C2 segment: Pain is around the eyes (periorbital) and ear.
C2-C3 segment: Pain around parietal and frontal regions.
C3-C4 segment: Pain in upper thoracic region and lateral cervical region.

The Brain Injury Association of America states that no pharmaceutical interventions have been found efficacious for this type of headache. Manual therapies may be used. Nerve injections, freeing the nerves, or even ablation may be recommended in persistent cases.

Craniomandibular Headache

This refers to head pain associated with the temporo-mandibular joint (TMJ) of the jaw. These may be very debilitating, causing difficulty with eating, talking or other movements of the jaw and mouth. Physical examination may reveal grinding sounds (crepitus). Bite blocks may be recommended and in persistent cases surgery may be recommended. Acupuncture may be helpful if of muscular origin.

Other Potential Non-vascular Etiologies
Anxiety: often bizarre pain, vise-like, vertex or general, emotional disturbance prominent
Post-traumatic: history of trauma, manifestations vary

EENT lesions: eyestrain, otitis, sinusitis, TMJ syndrome, manifestations vary
Brain tumor: mild to severe, localized initially then becomes generalized as tumor grows, intermittently persistent; slowly progressive weakness, convulsions, visual changes, aphasia, vomiting, mental changes; better or worse with postural changes
B*rain abscess:* history of EENT infection, lung abscess, rheumatic heart disease
Meningitis: constant, severe, generalized; fever, vomiting; preceding upper respiratory infection
S*ubdural hematoma:* trauma, changes in consciousness

Vascular
Intracerebral Hemorrhage
The result of a rupture of a vessel from hypertension or blood clot. Headaches tend to onset abruptly and severely. Neurological deficits steadily increase over time.

Subarachnoid Hemorrhage
An intercranial aneurysm, usually congenital, ruptures causing an abrupt, severe onset of headache. This may be accompanied by fainting, vomiting, dizziness, stiff neck, positive neurological testing signs

Toxic states: moderate, generalized, pulsating, constant; history of toxic exposure - infections, alcohol, uremia, lead, arsenic, etc.
H*ypertension:* throbbing, paroxysmal, occipital and vertex

Migraine Headaches
Migraines are considered a form of vascular headache caused by vasodilation of the large arteries of the brain. This dilation stretches the nerves that coil around the blood vessels, causing the nerves to release chemicals which cause inflammation, pain, and further vasodilation. This creates a feedback loop which magnifies the pain. 58% of returning soldiers who had post-traumatic headache experienced what were considered post-traumatic migraines.

Possible Etiology/Contributing Factors
-Family history
-More frequent in women [~3/4 of cases]
-Begins between ages of 10-30
-Often subside after age 50
-Vascular instability

-Headache from vasodilation
-Possible platelet abnormality – aggregation
-Prodrome may be due to vasoconstriction of cerebral blood vessels

Symptoms of Migraine Headaches
-Intense, throbbing or pounding pain that involves one temple or behind one eye and spreading outward. (Sometimes the pain is located in the forehead, around the eye, or at the back of the head).
-Heat, bright lights and excessive physical activity will tend to worsen symptoms.
-Tend to be unilateral (1/3 present bilaterally)
-Unilateral headaches typically change sides from one attack to the next.
-Unilateral headaches always occuring on the same side should see a primary care physician

Approximately 40-60% of cases the migraine may be preceded by prodrome that may include visual problems, partial paralysis, dizziness, mood swings/irritability, sleepiness, fatigue, depression or euphoria, yawning, craving sweet or salty foods. There may be a short period of depression, irritability, restlessness and anorexia. It is common for nausea, vomiting, diarrhea, facial pallor, cold and/or cyanotic hands or feet, and sensitivity to light and sound to accompany migraine headaches.

Due to light sensitivity, sufferers of migraines usually prefer to lie in a quiet, dark room during an attack. A typical attack lasts between 4 and 72 hours.

Types of Migraine Headaches
Classic migraines: Aura prior to headaches; usually more severe than common migraines.
Common migraine: accounts for 80% of migraines. No aura before a common migraine.

Migraine Aura
-Estimated 20% of migraines are associated with an aura. The most common auras are:
-Flashing, brightly colored lights in a zigzag pattern ("fortification spectra"), usually starting in the middle of the visual field and progressing outward
-A hole (scotoma) in the visual field ("blind spot").
-Some elderly sufferers may experience only visual aura without the headache
-Less common: pins-and-needles sensations in the hand and the arm on one side of the body or pins-and-needles sensations around the mouth and the nose on the same side.
-Auditory (hearing) hallucinations and abnormal tastes and smells.

Migraine Headache Treatment
Self-Care at Home:
-Using a cold compress to the area of pain
-Resting with pillows comfortably supporting the head or neck
-Resting in a room with little or no sensory stimulation (light, sound, odors)
-Withdrawing from stressful surroundings
-Sleeping
-Drinking a moderate amount of caffeine
-Nonsteroidal anti-inflammatory drugs (NSAIDS)
-Acetaminophen (Tylenol)
-Combination medications: include Excedrin Migraine, which contains acetaminophen and aspirin combined with caffeine.

Biomedical Treatment of Migraine Headaches:
Abortive:

-Combination of aspirin, acetaminophen, and caffeine
-Triptans, which specifically target serotonin
-Sumatriptan (Imitrex)
-Zolmitriptan (Zomig)
-Eletriptan (Relpax)
-Naratriptan (Amerge, Naramig)
-Rizatriptan (Maxalt)
-Frovatriptan (Frova)
-Almotriptan (Axert)

The following drugs are also specific in affecting serotonin, but they affect other brain chemicals. Occasionally, one of these drugs works when a triptan does not.
-Ergotamine tartrate (Cafergot)
-Dihydroergotamine (D.H.E. 45 Injection, Migranal Nasal Spray)
-Acetaminophen-isometheptene-dichloralphenazone (Midrin)

The following drugs are mainly used for nausea, but they sometimes have an abortive or preventive effect on headaches:
-Prochlorperazine (Compazine)
-Promethazine (Phenergan)

Weak narcotics; used primarily as a "backup" for the occasions when a specific drug does not work:
-Butalbital compound (Fioricet, Fiorinal)
-Acetaminophen and codeine (Tylenol with Codeine)

Preventive: considered if a patient has more than 1 migraine per week; the goal being to lessen the frequency and severity of the migraine attacks. Medications include:
-Antihypertensives:
-Beta-blockers (propranolol [Inderal])
-Calcium channel blockers (verapamil [Covera])
-Antidepressants:
       -Amitriptyline (Elavil)
       -Nortriptyline (Pamelor)
Anticonvulsants:
       -Gabapentin (Neurontin)
       -Valproic acid (Depakote)
       -Topiramate (Topamax)
-Antihistamines and anti-allergy drugs
       -Diphenhydramine (Benadryl)
       -Cyproheptadine (Periactin)

Other Therapies:
Botulinum toxin (BOTOX ®) injection

Cluster Headaches

Cluster headaches come in groups (clusters) lasting weeks or months, separated by pain-free periods of months or years. Pain typically happens once or twice daily, but some may experience pain more than twice daily. Each episode of pain generally lasts from 30 to 90 minutes with attacks generally happening around the same time every day and will often wake a person up when sleeping.

The pain is typically excruciating and located around or behind one eye. Some patients describe the pain as feeling like a hot poker in the eye. The affected eye may become red, inflamed, and watery. The nose on the affected side may become congested and runny. Unlike those with migraine headaches, people with cluster headaches tend to be restless. They often pace the floor, bang their heads against a wall, and can be driven to desperate measures. Cluster headaches are much more common in males than females.

Cluster Headaches Treatment
-Inhalation of high concentrations of oxygen
-Injection of tryptan medications
-Injection of lidocaine into the nostril
-Dihydroergotamine (DHE, Migranal), a vasoconstrictor
-Caffeine

99

Preventative cluster headache treatment considerations:
-Calcium channel blockers
        -Verapamil (Calan, Verelan, Verelan PM, Isoptin, Covera-HS)
        -Diltiazem (Cardizem, Dilacor, Tiazac)]
-Prednisone (Deltasone, Liquid Pred)

Antidepressant medications:
-Lithium (Eskalith, Lithobid)
-Valproic acid, divalproex (Depakote, Depakote ER, Depakene, Depacon)
-Topiramate (Topamax) (often used for seizure control)

Secondary Headaches

Causes of Secondary Headaches
The International Headache Society lists eight categories of secondary headache. A few examples in each category are noted (this is not a complete list):

-Head and neck trauma
-Blood vessel problems in the head and neck
-Stroke or transient ischemic attack (TIA)
-Arteriovenous malformations (AVM)
-Carotid artery inflammation
-Temporal arteritis (inflammation of the temporal artery)
-Non-blood vessel problems of the brain
-Brain tumors
-Seizures
-Idiopathic intracranial hypertension (once named pseudotumor cerebri): excessive cerebrospinal fluid pressure in the spinal canal.

-Medications and drugs (including withdrawal from those drugs)
-Infection
-Meningitis
-Encephalitis
-HIV/AIDS
-Systemic infections

-Post-craniectomy (Syndrome of Trephined): headache, dizziness, cognitive changes, etc. shrinking of the skin flap due to positional changes; treatment: cranioplasty to replace the bone flap

Problems of homeostasis:

-Hypertension
-Dehydration
-Hypothyroidism
-Renal dialysis

-Problems of the eyes, ears, nose throat, teeth and neck
-Psychiatric disorders
-Craniosacral Fluid Dynamics

Natural Treatment Approaches
-Acupuncture can often be a very effective treatment for many headache types
-Cold compress coated in a combination of lavender and peppermint essential oils.
-Liver/Kidney drainage if excess crystals present
-Treat underlying allergies
-Consider environmental allergens
-Cervical manipulation if appropriate
-Address any underling TMJ disorder symptoms
-Transcutaneous nerve stimulation (TENS)

-Biofeedback and relaxation therapy
-Guided imagery and relaxation

Dietary Considerations
-Avoid dietary amines: cheese, chocolate, beer, wine; allergens such as wheat or dairy
-Increase fiber and complex carbohydrates
-Blood sugar regulation as hypoglycemia can trigger

Orthomolecular Considerations
-Tryptophan
-5-HTP (100-200mg)
-Magnesium (Migraine) 400-800mg/day
-Vitamin B2 (Riboflavin) (400mg) (Migraine)
-Vitamin B6 (50-70mg)
-Quercetin – 500mg 15 minutes before eating
-Omega 3 fatty acids
-Niacin 100-400mg at first onset of symptoms

Phytotherapeutic Considerations
-Feverfew
-Butterbur
-Rosemary
-Majoram herbal tea
-Partenelle
-Meadow-sweet
-German Chamomile
-Ginger

Acupressure/Tapping Considerations
LI-4, GB-20, GB-40, GB-41,Yintang, Taiyang,

Acupuncture Research Studies
-A three-armed, parallel, randomized exploratory study of three military treatment facilities in the Washington, DC, metropolitan area of previously deployed Service members (18–69 years old) with mild-to-moderate TBI and headaches. Mean Headache Impact Test scores decreased in auricular acupuncture and traditional Chinese medicine groups while they increased slightly in the "usual care" only group from baseline to week 6 . Both acupuncture groups had sizable decreases in Numerical Rating Scale (Pain Best), compared to usual care.[1]

-Clinical signs of chronic headache (CH) disappeared markedly after three months of treatment with acupuncture. The amount of interleukin (IL)-1β, IL-6 and tumor necrosis factor-α (TNF-α) in LPS culture supernatant was significantly increased in the patients with CH compared to the healthy control group. Those cytokines came down toward the levels of the healthy group after treatment with acupuncture, although the levels still remained elevated. Significantly reduced plasma [cytokine] levels of TNF-α were also observed. "These data suggest that acupuncture treatment has an inhibitory effect on pro-inflammatory cytokine production in patients with [chronic headache]"[2]

-Before acupuncture treatment, the migraine without aura patients had significantly decreased functional connectivity in certain brain regions within the frontal and temporal lobe when compared with the healthy controls. After acupuncture treatment, brain regions showing decreased functional connectivity revealed significant reduction in migraine patients compared to before acupuncture treatment. Conclusions: Acupuncture treatment could increase the functional connectivity of brain regions in the intrinsic decreased brain networks in migraines without aura.[3]

-A review of studies found acupuncture may positively influence not just dynamic, but also static cerebral autoregulation during the interictal phase depending on the intervals between sessions of acupuncture as dose units. "Point-through-point" needling (at angles connecting acupoints) were found to possibly be clinically superior to standard acupuncture, thus needling angles may affect treatment effectiveness. [4]

Chapter 10
Fatigue

Fatigue is one of the most common symptoms following a head injury. It can span all levels of injury severity and can persist for many years in those with moderate-to-severity injuries. Fatigue is defined as "The awareness of a decreased capacity for physical and/or mental activity due to an imbalance in the availability, utilization, and/or restoration of resources needed to perform activity".

Many people who have sustained a brain injury experience a slowing down in their ability to process information and have difficulties with attention, memory and executive function (explored in later chapters). This can make mentally demanding tasks more daunting and draining. Studying may be difficult, energy for social interactions, and engagement in leisure activities may be affected. This can cause isolation and confinement at home which may turn to depression, even further exacerbating fatigue. This may impact major life activities or employment.

Much like headaches, fatigue can be primary or secondary in nature. Secondary fatigue may be a result of chronic pain, sleep difficulties, stress, or a poor overall quality of life. Depression and anxiety can also play into self-reported fatigue. Primary fatigue can be the result of diffuse brain injury as well as injury to the brain centers that controll arousal, attention and response speed. These may include the ascending reticulating activating system, limbic system, anterior cingulate, middle frontal lobe, and basal ganglia.

It has also been proposed that fatigue might result from hormonal dysregulation as a result of the injury. Growth hormone deficiency is common following a brain injury with studies showing as high as a 60% occurrence rate and is believed to be associated with fatigue. Others have proposed a connection between hypothalamic injury and fatigue following a brain injury.

Physiological Fatigue vs. Psychological Fatigue
Physiological fatigue can be caused by depletion of energy, hormones, neurotransmitters and/or a reduction in neural connections due to injury. Fatigue stemming from the peripheral nervous system can be assessed using motor tasks such as testing grip strength, thumb pressing or finger tapping speed, as these are unlikely to be affected by injury to the central nervous system.

Psychological fatigue is a state relating to reduced motivation, prolonged mental activity, or boredom resulting from chronic stress, anxiety, or depression. As all of these factors may be in play after a brain injury, psychological fatigue is an important factor to consider.

Fatigue can be addressed using natural approaches by generally tonifying any found deficiencies. Addressing stagnations present are also necessary. We will also look at a condition known as "chronic fatigue" to differentiate and explore approaching these issues.

Chronic Fatigue
Chronic fatigue syndrome, or chronic fatigue immune deficiency syndrome, is a

constellation of neurological, neuromuscular, and immunological abnormalities combined with cognitive impairments, disabling fatigue, and recurrent bouts of flu-like symptoms

Etiology and Symptoms
Unknown. Viral infection is strongly suspected, with 85% of sufferers experiencing an initial acute onset of flu-like symptoms such as mild fever, sore throat, tender lymph nodes, chills, and fatigue with minimal exertion.

This is then followed by symptoms such as:
-muscle pains (myalgia)
-joint pains
-sleep disorders
-headaches
-hyper or hyposensitivities
-cognitive disorders: spacial disorientation, short-term memory loss
-disabling fatigue and malaise
-depression, anxiety, irritability and/or confusion
-fluctuations in weight
-abdominal pain
-nausea and/or vomiting

Patients with this condition also often have a history of multiple allergies. Most patients are between 25-40 years of age.

Biomedical Diagnosis
There are no absolute clinical indicators or laboratory tests confirming this diagnosis. It is diagnosed primarily by presenting symptoms and history

Differential Diagnosis:
-Lupus
-Rheumatoid Arthritis
-Fibromyalgia

Biomedical Treatment
There is no specific biomedical treatment for chronic fatigue. It's current treatment is based on the management of symptoms.
For sleep: tricyclic depressants, seritonin reuptake inhibitors, benzodiazepine, clonazepam
For headache: NSAIDS (tension headache), calcium channel blockers (migraine)
For myalgias/arthralgias: muscle relaxants, NSAIDS, clonazepam
For candidiasis: ketoconazole (Nizoral), fluconazole (Diflucan)
For depression: anti-depressants
For fatigue: buproprion (Wellbutrin) and intramuscular B12 injections

Natural Treatment Approaches
Lifestyle Considerations
-Regulating and maintaining sleep is a very important component to fatigue after a brain

injury as the body needs plenty of rest to allow for the healing process
-Identify and remove causes of stress or learn to accept it if can't be changed
-Planning tools (calendars and alarms) to help the management of rest periods and naps on a regular basis. Try to limit naps to no more than 30 minutes at a time during the morning and early afternoon
-Do not resume activities faster than the management of fatigue allows
-Start with simple tasks, and gradually attempt more tasks as fatigue becomes manageable
-If necessary break every 5-10 minutes from an activity or exercise to avoid fatigue
-Use of a wheelchair or other assistive aid during trips, appointments, or visits may help prevent exhaustion
-Manage energy used up during appointments and visits and plan accordingly so as not to wear oneself out

Dietary Considerations
-Stabilize glucose levels
-Eat frequent meals (every 2-3 hr.) in glycemic healthy range for the individual
-Eat a protein and healthy fatty acid rich breakfast
-Don't wait until hungry, eat regularly to maintain a regular nutritional intake
-Nuts/seeds/eggs/ jerky (low sugar)
-Avoid fruit juice and carrot juice and junk food
-Veggies, meat
–high quality, grass fed, whole grains

Avoid:
-Concentrated simple sugars, caffeine, nicotine, alcohol, allergies, trans fats, omega-6 fatty acids (inhibits steroid synthesis, and disrupts normal anti-inflammatory cytokines), Artificial sweeteners (blocks conversion of phenylalanine to tyrosine, affecting catecholamine synthesis in adrenal medulla).

Somatic and Mindbody Considerations
-Stress reduction techniques
-Meditation
-Yoga
-Positive mental image
-Sedona technique
-Contract muscles and relax
-Exercise in aerobic range, No overtraining. Weight lifting, Yoga

Orthomolecular Considerations
-Omega 3 Fatty Acids
-B Vitamins
-Vitamin C (3000mg)
-Vitamin E (200-400 IU/day)
-Magnesium
-L-Carnitine (3000-4000mg)
-Phosphatidyl serine (affects cortisol)
-Sulfer amino acids, milk thistle: detox support
-Royal Jelly
-Cordyceps

Phytotherapeutic Considerations
-Astragalus (Huang Qi)
-Siberian Ginseng
-Codonopsis (Dang Shen)
-Ashwaghanda
-Rhodiola
-Licorice Root
-Panax Ginseng
-Maca
-Holy Basil

Acupressure/Tapping Considerations
ST-36, SP-6, CV-6, LI-10

Acupuncture Research Studies
-One hundred patients with chronic fatigue syndrome were randomly assigned to two groups of acupuncture in Qi Huang point [eight acupuncture needles in a 0.5 inch radius around the navel at 45 degree angles forming a complete circle] and the control group with routine therapy of acupuncture. Both groups received acupuncture for 30 minutes once every 3 days,10 times for 1 course, treatments lasting for 2 courses. Fatigue scale-14(FS-14) and self-rating depression scale (SDS) were used to evaluate the patients before and after treatment Scores after treatment were significantly lower than those before treatment in two groups, acupuncture in Qi Huang point of Chuang Medicine was shown to have better effects on chronic fatigue symptom.[2]

-47 cancer patients with moderate-severe fatigue were treated. Significant improvements were found with regards to General fatigue ($P < 0.001$), Physical fatigue ($P = 0.016$), Activity ($p = 0.004$) and Motivation ($P = 0.024$). At the end of the intervention, there was a 36% improvement in fatigue levels in the acupuncture group, while the acupressure group improved by 19% and the sham acupressure by 0.6%.[3]

-128 individuals with post-stroke fatigue where either given pharmaceuticals or electroacupuncture (EA) with cupping. Findings showed the effective rate of EA + cupping group was "obviously higher than that of medication group" and that the acupuncture plus cupping over the lower back "can effectively relieve fatigue of post-stroke patients, and its therapeutic effect is superior to medication." [4]

Chapter 11
Dizziness and the Vestibular System

Dizziness following a brain injury can be a common hindrance that can stem from changes or damage to the visual or vestibular system. Middle-aged and older individuals are at higher risk of more severe cases of dizziness and vertigo resulting in stroke. Hence, prevention and prompt treatment of dizziness and vertigo in older patients is very important. Given the wide range of impact it can have, visual system concerns will be discussed in a separate chapter later in this text. Here we will explore vestibular system dysfunction.

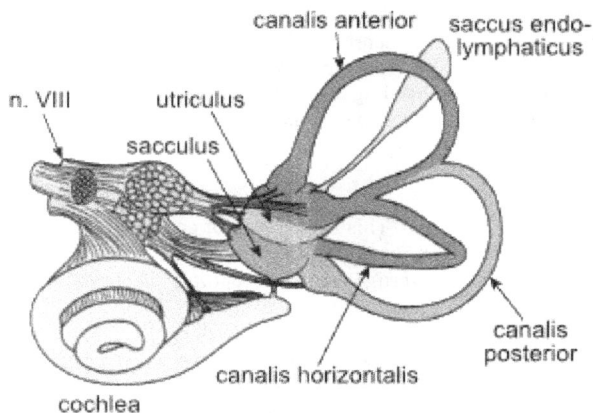

A variety of vestibular conditions may occur following a brain injury. These include:
Labyinthine Concussion (Unilateral Vestibular Hypofunction) – This is typically the result of trauma and bleed into the labyrinth. Symptoms may include:
-Dizziness
-Unilateral involuntary eye movements (nystagmus)
-Postural instability
-Balance loss or vision seeming to oscillate, blur or periodically jump (oscillopsia) with rotation of the head
Most cases (nearly 95%) improve from this condition within 6 months of injury.

Post-traumatic Meniere's Disease – Often the result of scarring and intermittent fluid build-up that impacts the pressure within the endolymphatic system which are known as hydrops. This can occur both shortly after or a while following an injury. Symptoms include:
-Intermittent bouts of dizziness (key diagnostic history)
-Low tone hearing loss with or without dizziness.
The membrane may rupture, worsening symptoms.

Vestibular Migraine – This may or may not be associated with a headache. Symptoms include:

-Episodic spinning dizziness lasting a few minutes, occurring multiple times within a month
-Light sensitivity (photophobia)
-Hearing loss and tinnitus may also be present

Basilar Skull Fracture – At the time of injury bleeding or leakage of cerebrospinal fluid into the ear can cause severe imbalance or dizziness. Medical observation or surgery are the commonly accepted medical treatment for this condition.

Perilymphatic fistula – This is an instance of perilymph leakage which causes abnormal communication between the inner and middle ear. Symptoms may include:
-Dizziness or loss of balance while blowing one's nose with eyes closed
-High tone hearing loss and increased dizziness with exposure to loud sounds
Minor surgery is the primary form of treatment.

Benign Paroxysmal Positioning Vertigo – This is the result of crystals in the semicircular canals being out of place or having debris attached to them. Symptoms include:
-Possible sensation of spinning with certain movements without hearing loss. These may include rolling in one direction, bending over, or changing positions while in bed.
A Dix-Hallpike movement test is used to diagnose this condition, making note of nystagmus or signs of dizziness with provoking positions. The repositioning maneuver can at times fully alleviate symptoms.

Bilateral Vestibular Hypofunction – This is the result of posture and gait abnormalities as well as difficulty focusing with movements of the head. Due to both sides of the vestibular system being affected, nausea or vertigo are rarely reported. These individuals may require assistive devices

Central Vertigo – This may be the result of trauma to the sensory inputs in the cervical spine or due to a vertebrobasilar insufficiency. Dizziness will be persistent as well as possibly coupled by the following symptoms based on the brain regions injured and whether it affects central or peripheral nerves:

Central Nerves Affected	-Abnormal eye movements (saccades, smooth pursuits) -Rare hearing loss (unless due to other trauma) -Double vision (Diplopia) -Tendency to fall to one side (Lateropulsion) -Vertigo symptoms that can't be fixed by stabilizing vision -Pendular nystagmus with eyes equal -Vertical involuntary eye movements (nystagmus) continues after changes in position
Peripheral Nerves Affected	-Normal eye movement screen -Involuntary eye movement (nystagmus) with positional testing -Possible tinnitus, fullness in ears, or insidious hearing loss that may recover -Very intense acute vertigo in which visual fixation can help -Jerk nystagmus present (both fast and slow phases) -Spontaneous horizontal nystagmus (generally resolves in ~1 week or less)

Diagnostic Testing
A physiatrist examination may be done to determine the nature of vestibular dysfunction. Possible diagnostics include:
-Audiogram
-Video or electronystagmography (VNG/ENG)
-Electrocochleography (EcoG)
-Platform Posturography
-MRI
-MRA/MRV
-CT
-Arteriography

Biomedical Approaches
-Meclizine hydrochloride (Antivert)
-Scopolamine transdermal patch (Transderm-Scop)
-Promethazine hydrochloride (Phenergan)
-Metoclopramie (Reglan)
-Odansetron (Zofran)

-Diazepam (Valium)
-Lorazepan (Ativan)
-Clonazepam (Klonopin)
-Prednisone (Deltasone, Liquid Pred, Sterapred)

Emerging Treatment Methods – virtual reality
Balance deficits can be very common following a TBI and can cause physical limitations that can be both difficult to deal with and frustrating. It has been estimated that almost all of those admitted to an inpatient rehab environment with a TBI have some form of balance impairment. An emerging evidence-based treatment for those with neurogenic balance impairment is the use of virtual reality systems that allow them to view a virtual environment and dynamically respond and interact with it in real time.

Natural Treatment Approaches
Lifestyle Considerations
-Decrease consumption of rich foods and alcohol
-Abstain from hot, spicy foods
-Stress management / controlling the emotions
-Engage in appropriate physical exercise

Orthomolecular Considerations
-Vitamin B6
-Vitamin C
-Vitamin D
-Coenzyme Q10

Phytotherapeutic Consdierations
-Ginkgo Biloba
-Gastrodia (Tian Ma)

-Chinese herbal supplementation (Formulations determined by professional)

Acupressure/Tapping Considerations
TW-2, TW-3, TW-17, GB-12

Acupuncture Research Studies
-60 recruited patients in an emergency room. The variation of Visual Analog Scale demonstrated a significant decrease between two groups after two different durations: 30 mins and 7 days. Heart rate variability also showed a significant increase in high frequency (HF) in the acupuncture group. No adverse event was reported in this study. It was concluded "Acupuncture demonstrates a significant immediate effect in reducing discomforts and VAS [visual analog scale] of both dizziness and vertigo. This study provides clinical evidence on the efficacy and safety of acupuncture to treat dizziness and vertigo in the emergency department."[1]

-A summary of the literature showed that acupuncture in the treatment of cervical vertigo acts to dilate blood vessels, diminish vessel resistance and increase blood flow, hence to improve micro-circulation and oxygen supply to the brain[2]

-The investigation at Jianghan University employed a combination of electroacupuncture and ultrasound for the treatment of vertigo focusing on efficacy for the treatment of vertigo due to posterior circulation ischemia from dysfunction of the vertebrobasilar arterial system. This combination achieved a 94.29% total effective rate. As a stand alone therapy, electroacupuncture achieved a 68.57% total effective rate. Using only ultrasound, the researchers achieved a 71.43% total effective rate. Based on the data, the researchers conclude that a combination of electroacupuncture and ultrasound therapies achieves superior patient outcomes over using either modality alone.[3]

Chapter 12
Tinnitus

Tinnitus is a ringing, buzzing, roaring, whistling or hissing sound that seems to originate from within the ear or head. It is a commonly occurring symptom following a TBI. The noise may be constant or intermittent and vary in pitch from a low roar to a high squeal. It may be heard in one or both ears. Tinnitus is not a single disease, but rather a symptom of another underlying condition. Heavy use of antibiotics or aspirin can also cause tinnitus to occur.

In many cases (though not all) tinnitus itself is not a serious problem, but rather a nuisance. Much of the literature on brain injury makes mention of it but does not tend to elaborate greatly. Statistics on experiencing some form of hearing loss have rates as high as 44% in cases not caused by a blast injury and 62% in cases of blast injuries[1].

This can have an impact on one's means of communicating with others. Hearing loss can go unnoticed however, and be attributed to confusion or deficits in attention and memory. An assessment by an audiologist may be needed to gauge severity of hearing loss and possible causes.

Until fairly recently, most accounts of tinnitus in textbooks said it was exclusively due to ear damage which could not be fixed. More recent research, however, suggests that with the majority of cases of tinnitus there are no definable physical abnormalities within the ear. Researchers using positron emission tomography (PET scan) to view the brain activity of people with tinnitus have been able to show that these phantom auditory sensations originated somewhere *within the brain*, not within the ear. It seems, therefore, that tinnitus can be something akin to a phantom limb pain or focal dystonia, where symptoms result from aberrant neural activity in the brain.[2] Muscle tension in the neck and around the skull can also affect the inner ear and cause tinnitus.

Possible Etiology
-Traumatic (e.g., injury to head and neck)
-Age-related (a.k.a. presbycusis)
-Occupational/Noise-induced
-Toxic (e.g., aminoglycoside antibiotics, aspirin)
-Congenital (e.g., otosclerosis)
-Infectious (e.g. otitis media)
-Cardiovascular (a.k.a. Pulsatile Tinnitus)
-Atherosclerosis
-Hypertension
-Turbulent blood flow
-Arteriovenous malformation
-Head and neck tumors
-Other (physical obstruction such as earwax, Meniere's disease, acoustic neuroma)

Biomedical Treatment
There are, as yet, no cures for tinnitus but there are several treatments currently used to

produce relief:
-Acoustic Therapy: the addition or enhancement of external sounds that can reduce the perception of tinnitus using any of the following:
1) sound generators that are worn in the ears
2) hearing aids;
3) tapes, CDs, and bedside units that can help with sleep or concentration
4) pillows embedded with small speakers that can plug into any tape, CD, or sound generation machine

-Pharmaceutical: tricyclic antidepressants such as amitriptyline, nortriptyline, gabapentin (Neurontin), and acamprosate (Campral)
-Surgical Intervention

Clinical Notes:
-Children are less likely to complain of tinnitus or loss of hearing, but will complain of earache

Natural Treatment Approaches
-Counseling
-Tinnitus Retraining Therapy (TRT): a combination of low level, broad-band noise and counseling to habituate to the tinnitus. That is, the individual becomes no longer aware of their tinnitus, except when they focus their attention on it, and even then tinnitus is not annoying or bothersome.[3]

Dietary Considerations:
eating principles:
-low fat diet, low sugar, high complex carbohydrates
-protein 12-15% diet
-low cholesterol/cholesterol foods
-vegetarian cleansing diet or short fasts

chronic:
-elimination/rotation diet, rotation diet, rotation diet expanded

-Foods that tonify the Kidney,: black sesame seeds, black beans, celery, oyster shells, pearl barley, adzuki beans, black jujube, yams, lotus seed, chestnuts, grapes

- liver-cleansing foods: beets, carrots, artichokes, lemons, parsnips, dandelion greens, watercress, burdock root, chrysanthemum flowers and tea

avoid: stimulating foods, hot, spicy foods, rich foods, coffee, alcohol

Orthomolecular Considerations
- Oral Magnesium (aspartate) low levels of magnesium (~200mg) are associated with noise-induced hearing loss; supplementation with magnesium has been shown to prevent noise-induced hearing loss[5]
- Cobalamin (B12) - Individuals with tinnitus and noise-induced hearing loss have demonstrated significant vitamin B-12 deficiency. Determination of vitamin B12 status in

individuals with tinnitus and noise-induced hearing loss is warranted. If low, supplement with 2,000 mcg daily for 1 month, followed by 1,000 mcg daily thereafter (sublingual methylcobalamin is preferred form). Take with folic acid.

Phytotherapeutic Considerations
-Oats: nerve tonic
-Black Cohosh: vertigo from auditory tinnitus
-Ginkgo biloba (standardized extract): 40 milligrams, 3 times a day. It may take 3 months or more of continued use
-Goldenseal: catarrhal deafness and tinnitus
-St. John's Wort: internally; oil, locally in the ear canal
-Catsfoot: tinnitus aurium
-Mullein
-Periwinkle[6, 7]
-Prickly Ash: circulatory stimulant
-Cordyceps (Dong Chong Xia Cao)
-Kudzu Root (Ge Gen)
-Fu Ti (He Shou Wu)
-Gentian Root (Long Dan Cao)
-Oyster Shell (Mu Li)

Acupressure/Tapping Considerations
TW-2. TW-3, GB-8, GB-20, TW-17

-TW-17 and GB-20 can be a potent combination and can release the musculature in the occipital region. So much so that stimulation with lift-thrust technique or twisting the needle can sometimes bring the volume of ringing down in real time almost like a volume knob on a stereo. Taking time to find the proper angle and position can at times provide significant relief to the individual.

Acupuncture Research Studies:
-"Two separate groups were tested with the acupuncture point prescriptions. Both groups had an acupuncture needle retention time of thirty minutes. Acupuncture was conducted once per day for a grand total of eighteen acupuncture treatments. The first set of acupuncture points outperformed the second set by 30% with a total effective rate of 80%... A total of 64.17% patients fully recovered, 14.71% had significant improvements, 11.76% had slight improvements, and 8.82% had no improvements. The total effective rate was 91.18%. The researchers concluded that acupuncture combined with ginger moxibustion is effective for the treatment of intractable tinnitus. The researchers note that widespread adoption of this clinical treatment protocol is warranted based on the significant rate of positive patient outcomes." [8]

- 50 patients (46 males, 4 females) suffering from tinnitus were were randomly assigned to three groups: a manual acupuncture group (MA), an electrical acupuncture group (EA), and a placebo group (PL). The frequency of tinnitus occurrence, tinnitus intensity, and reduction of life quality were recorded before treatment (Baseline), after 6 treatments (After-Treatment), and 1 month after the completion of treatment (1-Month-After). Standard audiometric tests were conducted on each patient at Baseline and After-Treatment. 6

113

treatments were performed at weekly intervals. The frequency of tinnitus occurrence and the tinnitus loudness were significantly decreased After-Treatment compared with Baseline in the EA group. Life quality was improved After-Treatment and at 1-Month-After compared with Baseline in both MA and EA groups. However, no significant differences were detected among the three groups with the audiogram not showing any significant changes after treatment in either group ($P > 0.091$). The overall subjective evaluation indicated significant improvements after-treatment compared with baseline in both MA and EA groups. After-Treatment subjective evaluation was significantly better in the EA group compared with either the MA or PL group.[9]

-90 cases of nervous tinnitus were randomly divided evenly into 3 groups, 30 cases in each group. The acupuncture group were treated with acupuncture at cervical Jiaji (EX-B 2), 20 min each session, once a day, 10 sessions constituting one course. The Chinese herbs group was treated with modified Buzhong Yiqi Decoction (decocted in water), one dose each day, 10 doses constituting one course; the western medicine group with bandazol, Dextran 40, Danshen tablet, and vitamin B12, 10 days constituting one course. After 3 courses, the therapeutic effects were evaluated finding the effective rates in the 3 groups were 73.3%, 40.0% and 33.3%, respectively, with significant differences among the 3 groups. It was concluded " Acupuncture has obvious therapeutic effect on nervous tinnitus, and acupuncture at cervical Jiaji (EX-B 2) is an effective therapy for nervous tinnitus, and its therapeutic effect is better than those of Chinese herbs and western medicine."[10]

Chapter 13
Nausea and Vomiting

Nausea can often occur after a brain injury. This is particularly true immediately following a mild TBI. In cases where other symptoms are present or become chronic such as headaches, migraines, dizziness/vertigo, dysphagia, visual disturbances, and seizures; nausea may accompany them as a secondary problem. Because nausea generally accompanies these other conditions, it is rarely addressed or studied on it's own and results in a lack of available statistics. Because at times nausea and/or vomiting can become severe enough to warrant specific treatment, it is worth including natural approaches to addressing it.

Terminology
Vomiting (emesis): oral expulsion of gastrointestinal contents
Regurgitation: Effortless passage of gastric contents into the mouth
Retching: The muscular movements without actual vomiting (ie, "dry heaves")
Nausea: A feeling of the need to vomit but does not necessarily do so
Dyspepsia: "upset stomach", includes burning, gnawing discomfort, bloating, or pain.

The vomiting center of the brain lies in the medulla oblongata and comprises the rutabaga formation and the nucleus of the tractus solitarius. When activated, motor pathways descend from this center and trigger vomiting. These pathways travel within the 5th, 7th, 9th, 10th, and 12th cranial nerves to the upper gastrointestinal tract. The vomiting center can be activated directly by irritants or indirectly following input from 4 principal areas: the gastrointestinal tract, cerebral cortex and thalamus, vestibular region, and the chemoreceptor trigger zone (CRTZ). Unlike other brain centers, it is not protected by the blood-brain barrier and is easily prone to irritants.

Before vomiting occurs, there may be a period of antiperistalsis, in which rhythmic contractions occur up the digestive tract instead of downward. Distention within these upper portions of the gastrointestinal tract then generates impulses to the vomiting center, where the actual act of vomiting is initiated. For this reason, an empty stomach does not preclude vomiting.

Biomedical Interventions
Antiemetic Drugs
Those that block acetylcholine and histamine appear most useful when vestibular triggers are suspected. Dopamine blockade targets the emetogenic influence of opioids in the vomiting center and CRTZ. Unfortunately, their ability to also block dopamine transmission in the basal ganglia can result in so-called extrapyramidal syndromes (EPSs) that include akathisia (restlessness) , parkinsonian symptoms, and tardive dyskinesia. The serotonin antagonists act not only in the vomiting center but within the GI tract, where surgical manipulation or many of the chemotherapeutic agents have a noxious influence. Anxiolytic medications are useful in cases where anticipatory anxiety is high.

Dopamine Antagonists
-Promethazine (Phenergan)

-Prochlorperazine (Compazine) are among the most commonly used antiemetics
-Metoclopramide (Reglan) has a prokinetic action on the upper digestive tract.
-Droperidol -May trigger tachyarrhythmia

5-HT3 (Serotonin) Blockers
The 5-HT3 (serotonin) antagonists were introduced initially to combat radiation and
chemotherapy-induced nausea and vomiting. This was due to chemotherapeutic agents
triggering serotonin release within the gastrointestinal wall.
-Ondansetron (Zofran).

Novel Agents
Drugs that block the neurokinin 1 (NK1) receptor have proven efficacy in chemotherapy-
induced nausea and vomiting. They are most effective in preventing delayed nausea and
generally are used in conjunction with 5-HT3 antagonists for this reason.
- Aprepitant (Emend)
-Cannabinols such as tetrahydrocannabinol found in marijuana and dronabinol (Marinol), a
synthetic derivative, have proven efficacy for chemotherapy-induced nausea and vomiting.
-Glucocorticoids:
-Dexamethasone: mechanism unknown but may suppress production of inflammatory
autacoids that may somehow potentiate known vomiting pathways within the vomiting
center. Benefit is limited to prophylactic regimens.

Potential Contributing Factors

-Variations in blood calcium levels
-Potassium Excess
-Zinc toxicity
-Biotin toxicity
-Manganese excess
-Niacin toxicity
-Iodine toxicity
-Selenium excess

Clinical Notes
- Referral to an acute-care medical facility is strongly recommended if dehydration due to
severe vomiting is evident. Referral is also necessary if there is projectile vomiting with
blood in the vomit, high fever, severe headache, irritability, lethargy or unconsciousness.

Natural Treatment Approaches

Lifestyle Considerations
-Identify and avoid odors or spices that trigger nausea
-Remove any environmental toxicity exposure
-Emotions of anger, fear, ambivalence, doubt, resentment, disgust, denial, or unresolved
conflict cause play a role and should be addressed, potentially with counseling

Dietary Considerations
-Avoid spicy meals, alcohol and fats
-Eat small, regular meals to prevent blood sugar from falling

-Drink plenty of fluids to avoid dehydration
-Fresh vegetables, especially green leafy vegetables, balanced proteins, fiber, complex carbohydrates

Orthomolecular Considerations
-Vitamin B6
-Vitamin C

Phytotherapeutic Considerations
-Ginger (Gan Jiang) can often be effective for nausea
-Peppermint
-Chamomile

Acupressure/Tapping Considerations
PC-6, ST-36, Yintang, Ear: stomach, shenmen

- "Sea Bands" or similar products that apply pressure over the acupuncture point PC-6 may be a useful and accessible option for some.

Acupuncture Research Studies:
- Stimulation of point PC-6 has been studied and been found significantly effective in cases of Post-operative Nausea and Vomiting(PONV). Acupuncture may reduce nausea and vomiting via endogenous beta-endorphin release in the cerebrospinal fluid or a change in serotonin transmission via activation of serotonergic and noradrenergic fibers. The exact mechanisms have yet to be established. "Electroacupuncture at this point is also effective for postoperative nausea. "Stimulation of P 6 has been shown to be as effective as pharmacological treatment for PONV with ondansetron in both adults and children."[2]

117

118

Chapter 14
Dysphagia

Dysphasia is a disturbance in the ability to swallow. It can occur for many reasons including motor control impairment, weakness of facial, masticatory, pharyngeal or laryngo-esophageal muscles, a loss of coordination between breathing and muscle function, and changes in sensory processing. The digestive system involves regulation from the hypothalamus through the parasympathetic and sympathetic nervous systems. The digestive tract and the higher brain structures also regulate nutritional intake. Either sensory or motor neural deficits can lead to dysphagia. Isolated cranial nerve deficits can include the facial nerve (CN VII), glossopharyngeal nerve (CN IX), vagus nerve (CN X), and hypoglossal nerve (CN XII).

Diagnostic Testing
Diagnostically a modified barium swallow test will be done by a radiologist or physiatrist and speech language pathologist.
-Videofluoroscopic Swallowing Study (VFSS) is a barium swallowing exam using real-time x-rays to see the bolus flow and structural movements of the digestive tract. This is particularly helpful in determining improvements for swallowing food and developing strategies toward restoring nutritional intake.

-Water-swallowing test (WST) is an exam that detects aspiration and is useful in developing strategies to prevent pneumonia. The WST uses drinking to assess successful swallows, swallowing speed, time to swallow, coughing, choking, or otherwise drinking.

After a brain injury someone may require being intubated for a period of time. A feeding tube will provide both hydration and calories via the tube surgically implanted into either the stomach (gastrostomy) or the small intestine (jejunostomy). These require nurses, trained staff or family to assure proper administration and prevent risks of aspiration or over distention. There are four levels of diet abilities in dysphagia. The level of lowest functionability is dysphagia pureed, followed by dysphagia mechanically altered, dysphagia advanced and finally regular diet, with each level allowing for consumption of more complex foods.

LEVEL	DYSPHAGIA SEVERITY	DESCRIPTION
Level 1 Dysphagia Pureed	Moderate to Severe	Consists of pureed, cohesive foods with a consistency close to pudding.
Level 2 Dysphagia Mechanically Altered	Mild to Moderate and/or pharyngeal dysphagia	All foods from level one, plus foods that are moist, soft textured, and easily form a bolus. Food pieces no larger than ¼ inch. Some chewing ability
Level 3 Dysphagia	Mild	This level includes most textures except hard, sticky or crunchy foods. This level

Advanced		includes soft foods that require chewing
Level 4 Regular Diet	N/A	All foods are tolerated

There are also four levels of liquid viscosity tolerated:

LEVEL	DESCRIPTION
Thin	No alteration
Nectar-like	Slightly thicker than water, the consistency of un-set gelatin
Honey-like	A liquid with the consistency of honey
Spoon-thick	A liquid with the consistency of pudding

Therapeutic Interventions
-Cold stimulation
-Practicing of swallowing
-Breath hold techniques
-Voicing exercises
-Throat contraction exercises
-Throat lifting exercises
-Face and lips muscle functional training
Many of these are provided or worked with a Speech-Language Pathologist

Other possible concerns
Gastrointestinal concerns following a brain injury include hyperphasia (excessive eating), coughing while eating, dehydration, anorexia (disinterest or loss of appetite) and gastroesophageal reflux disease (GERD).

Biomedical Approaches
Biomedical medications for GERD include Prilosec, Protonix, Zantac, Pepcid and Reglan. Though blocking acid production and reflux, these may increase the risk of cognitive changes or impairment

The detrimental effects of dysphagia can have a significant impact. The metabolic needs of the individual increases significantly following a moderate-to-severe brain injury as the body requires these resources to heal the brain. This is required for the health of all cells, cognitive function, and overall recovery. The Congress of Neurological Surgeons states that a person will need at least 40% more calories in the acute phase of recovery than prior to the injury. This increases in relation to the severity of the injury and the effects can at times persist indefinitely.

Natural Treatment Approaches

Phytotherapeutic Considerations
-Tan Xiang (White Sandalwood)
-Fig

-Blackcurrant
-Silver Linden

Acupuncture Point Considerations
Local:
SI-17, CV-17, CV-22, CV-23, CV-24, ST-4, LI-18

Distal Point and their relevant clinical indications:
        PC-8 "Inability To Swallow Food "
        GB-39 "Occlusion of the throat with oppressive feeling, difficulties
                in swallowing "
        TW-7 "Tongue paralyzed, cannot swallow (glosso-labio-pharyngeal paralysis "
        BL-17 "Difficulty swallowing"
        BL-21 "Dysphagia"
        LI-11 "Dysphagia"

Points correlating to potentially affected cranial nerves according to YNSA:
        -Facial nerve (CN VII)
        -Glossopharyngeal nerve (CN IX)
        -Vagus nerve (CN X)
        -Hypoglossal nerve (CN XII)

Acupuncture Research Studies
- A Meta-analysis of 6 enrolled trials showed that the acupuncture group had a better therapeutic effect on dysphagia after stroke than the control group.[1]

-*Tongguan Liqiao* acupuncture therapy has been shown to effectively treat dysphagia after stroke-based pseudobulbar paralysis. Sixty-four patients with dysphagia following brainstem infarction were divided into groups according to infarction location: medulla, midbrain and pons, and a multiple cerebral infarction group according to MRI results. Acupuncture was done at PC-6, GV-26, SP-6, GB-20, GB-12, TW-17 twice daily (30 minute retention time) for 28 days. The total efficacy rate was 92.2% after treatment, and was most obvious in patients with medulla oblongata infarction (95.9%). These findings suggest that *Tongguan Liqiao* acupuncture therapy can repair the connection of upper motor neurons to the medulla oblongata motor nucleus, promote the recovery of brainstem infarction, and improve patient's swallowing ability and quality of life.[2]

-Another metaanalysis of literature showed treatments duration averaging 24.8 in length with an average total effective rate was 91.2%. In these CV-23, GB-20, GV-16 and TW-17 were the most commonly used acupoints from the regular meridians, while Jinjin (EX-HN 12) and Yuye (EX-HN 13) were the most commonly used extraordinary acupoints.[4]

-A total of 90 dysphagia patients with craniocerebral injuries participated. A total of 43 patients were cases with cerebral infarction, 24 cases with cerebral hemorrhage, 13 cases with traumatic injury, and 10 other cases of CCI. They were randomly split into 3 groups of rehabilitation exercises only, rehabilitation exercises with additional neuromuscular electrical stimulation, and rehabilitation exercise with additional neuromuscular electrical stimulation and acupuncture. Acupuncture using points ST-7, ST-6, ST-4. HT-5, LI-4 were shown to have a significant benefit. [5,6]

Chapter 15
Seizures/Epilepsy

A seizure is defined as a sudden, brief attack of altered consciousness, motor activity, sensory phenomena, and/or inappropriate behavior. They can be recurrent or sudden occurrences and thought to involve an excessive discharge of neurons when a brief, strong surge of electrical activity affects part, or all of the brain. One in 10 adults are estimated to have a seizure at some point during their life. Each year 200,000 new cases of epilepsy are diagnosed. Incidences of seizure activity are higher in those under the age of 2 and over 65. 70% of these new cases have no apparent or known cause.

Seizures can last from a few seconds to a few minutes. They can have many symptoms - from convulsions and loss of consciousness to some less associated symptoms by the person experiencing them or by health care professionals. These may include blank staring, lip smacking, or jerking movements of arms and legs.

Post-traumatic seizures occur depending on the amount of time since the injury, severity of the injury, and the age of the individual at the time of trauma. Because of this, statistics range from a 4-53% incidence in individuals with brain injury. Young adults and military injuries tend to be at the greatest risk. Trauma is said to be responsible for 20% of cases of symptomatic epilepsy.

Epilepsy is unique in that it can recur suddenly and unexpectedly, which can lead to set backs, both physical and psychological, that can be detrimental to recovery. The more severe the injury, tissue damage, and bleeding are associated with a higher risk of epilepsy. 5% of individuals with a closed head injury have been shown to develop post-traumatic epilepsy, while those sustaining an open injury showed a 30-50% incidence.

Post-traumatic seizures and epilepsy can affect an individuals quality of life, employment ability, ability to drive, as well as increasing risk of further physical injury. This includes another head injury. Depression can occur alongside seizure activity as well as being a risk factor for developing epilepsy.

Etiology
Closed head injuries may involve diffuse axonal injury and neuronal shearing, focal hemorrhage and contusion. Penetrating injuries carry risk of bone fragments making their way into the cranial cavity. New scar tissue on the cortical surface may also form.

Early seizures may be due to metabolic changes such as edema, ischemia, or the release of toxic mediators in the damaged brain tissue.

Late post-traumatic seizures have been associated with iron deposition in the tissue due to hemoglobin breaking down and forming free radicals. This disrupts cell walls and causes cell death.

Seizure activity may also occur as a result of increased excitatory neurotransmitters (such as glutamate) while inhibitory neurotransmitters such as GABA become less.

Post-Traumatic Seizure Types
Immediate Post-traumatic Convulsions (IPTC)
This occurs within seconds of impact, involving a loss of consciousness and involuntary movements. These episodes are generally considered non-epileptic events and closer to fainting. This may start with a short period of body rigidity, followed jerking movements that last less than 2-3 minutes. Following the acute episode the person may experience an altered state of consciousness that tends to be associated with retrograde and anterograde amnesia. Most of the literature on IPTC is from observation of sports injuries and estimate them happening in 1 out of 70 concussions. Recurrent seizures are rare in cases of IPTC and thus rarely require anticonvulsant medications for prevention.

Early Post-Traumatic Seizures (ETPS)
These occur within the first 7 days following a head injury. 50% of convulsive EPTS occur within the first 24 hours of injury with 25% of cases occurring within the first hour. These can be found in mild as well as more severe TBI and has been reported to have an incidence of 2-10% in brain injuries. While statistics on non-convulsive EPTS have not been gathered, the Brain Injury Association of America states it may occur in as many as 5% of EPTS cases.

Late Post-Traumatic Seizures (LPTS)
These are seizures that occur more than one week following an injury. Onset generally happens within the first 18-24 months of the brain injury but has been reported many years later. Reported incidence of LPTS ranges anywhere from 1.9-50%. While an isolated seizure incidence is possible, most sources will use the term post-traumatic epilepsy interchangeably with LPTS as they carry a higher risk of epilepsy than other seizure types. Children were found to be less prone to LPTS, while those over 65 years of age seemed more at risk. The strongest risk factors for LPTS seem to be missile wounds, bilateral or multiple contusions, and multiple craniotomies.

Statis Epilepticus
This is a condition defined as greater than 30 minutes of continuous seizure activity or two or more events occurring without a full recovery of consciousness between episodes. This condition occurs within approximately 10% of individuals after an acute head injury. It is more commonly found within children. Confused states following a brain injury need to be distinguished from the possibility of

124

nonconvulsive statis epilepticus (NCSE). NCSE can involve a confusional state as well as bizarre behavior, sedation or stupor.

Biomedical Treatments
Prophylaxis/ Late Post-Traumatic Seizures

Antiepileptic Drug	Beneficial Effects	Potentially Harmful Effects
Barbiturates: e.g. Phenobarbital (Solfoton)	Anxiety, mood stabilization, sleep	Aggression, impaired cognition and attention, depression, irritability, sexual function and desire
Carbamazepine (Tegretol)	Aggression, mania, mood stabilization	Irritability, impaired attention
Ethosuximide (Zarontin)	Data not available	Aggression, confusion, depression, insomnia
Gabapentin (Neurontin)	Anxiety, insomnia, social phobia, mood stabilization	Irritability/agitation (usually in children with disabilities)
Lamotrigine (Lamictal)	Depression, mood stabilization, mania	Insomnia, irritability (usually in children with disabilities)
Levetiracetam (Keppra)	Data not available	Anxiety, depression, irritability (all appear more common in children), highest rate of psychiatric side effects (more common in those with psychiatric history)
Phenytoin (Dilatin)	Mania	Depression, impaired attention
Tiagabine (Gabitril)	Mania, mood stabilization	Depression, irritability
Topiramate (Topamax)	Binge eating, mania, mood stabilization, ethanol dependane	Depression, impaired cognition (word finding, memory) and attention, irritability
Valproate (Depakote)	Agitation, aggression, irritability, mania, mood stabilization	Depression
Zonisamide (Zonegran)	Mania	Aggression, emotional lability, irritability

Other possible pharmaceuticals
-Clonazepam (Klonopin)
-Primidone (Mysoline)
-Lacosamide (Vimpat)
-Rufinamide (Banzel)

-Diazepam (Valium)
-Lorazepam (Ativan)
-Oxcarbazepine (Trileptal)
-Pregabalin (Lyrica)

Statis Epilepticus
-Benzoidiapines
-Intravenous phenytoin or fosphenytoin
-Barbiturates
-Propofol
-Valproate

Other Possible Causes of Seizures
Sympomatic
-high fever, CNS infections, metabolic disturbances (hypoglycemia), toxic, hypoxia, tumors, congenital brain defects, cerebral edema, cerebral trauma, anaphylaxis, brain bleeds

Idiopathic
- 75% of all seizures occur in young adults
- before age 2 - developmental defects, metabolic disturbances, birth injury
- after age 25 - tumors, trauma
- focal brain disease can cause seizures at any age

Classifications
Generalized Seizure
Both hemispheres are affected . Loss of consciousness and motor function

absence (petit mal)	grand mal (tonic-clonic)	atonic (astatic, akinetic)
Generalized 10-30 second loss of consciousness with eye or muscle flutterings Stops activity and then resumes it after attack is over Often when sitting quietly Genetic Does not begin after age 20	Generalized Occasional aura Loss of consciousness Tonic-clonic contractions of muscles of extremities, trunk, head 2-5 minutes Postictal state - sleep, headache, muscle soreness	Brief, generalized Complete loss of muscle tone and consciousness Head drops, loss of posture, or sudden collapse. Protective headgear is sometimes used to protect head during falling. Tends to resist drug treatment
myoclonic	infantile spasms	febrile
Brief, quick jerks or clumsiness May be repetitive Occasionally involves only one arm or a foot. No loss of consciousness	Sudden flexion of arms and trunk with extension of legs Lasts a few seconds, several times daily Only in first 3 years of life Associated with developmental abnormalities	3 months to 5 yrs old High fever In 4% of all children - 2% of those Develop epilepsy

Partial Seizure
In partial seizures the electrical disturbance is limited to a specific region in one hemisphere of the brain. Partial seizures may spread to cause a generalized seizure. Partial seizures are the most common type of seizure experienced by people with epilepsy. Virtually any movement, sensory, or emotional symptom can occur as part of a partial seizure, including complex visual or auditory hallucinations.

Simple partial (focal)
-Specific sensory, motor, without loss of consciousness - aura is one

Jacksonian seizure
-Focal symptoms begin in hand or foot and march up extremity
-May be local or proceed to generalized seizure

Complex partial (psychomotor)
-1-2 minute loss of contact with surroundings: purposeless movements, unintelligible sounds, staggering
-No understanding
-Structural pathology

Partial Seizure Manifestations	
Frontal Lobe	Brain sensations, autonomic sensations, involuntary movement, forced or obscure thoughts or actions
Frontal Complex (Orbital or Mesial)	Often occur at night, strong expression: screaming or cursing, intense thrashing movements, pelvic thrusting, complex automatisms (bicycling, boxing etc), irregular movements
Temporal Lobe (Mesial)	Fear (amygdala involvement), sensation of somebody behind them, deja vu, jamais vu, rising epigastric sensation, autonomic symptoms (flushing, increased heart rate, hypertension, peristalsis, respiratory arrest, sweating, urinary incontinence, goosebumps), vomiting (right lobe), illusions, visual hallucinations, olfactory hallucinations (foul odor via basal forebrain) depersonalization, derealization
Temporal Lobe (Lateral)	Aphasia, vertigo, simple auditory hallucinations
Parietal Lobe	Simple or complex sensory phenomena, pain (rare)
Occipital Lobe	Simple or complex visual hallucinations (less experiental than temporal hallucinations), vomiting

Psychic Phenomena During Partial Seizures	
Cognitive	"Dreamy state", derealization, depersonalization, dissociation, mystical/religious experiences, forced thinking, altered speed of thoughts, distortion of time, distortion of body image

Dysphasic	Speech arrest, nonfluent speech, paraphasias, comprehension deficit, repetitive utterances, dyslexia, agraphia
Dysmnesic	Deja Vu, jamais vu, selective memory impairment, forced recollection
Affective	Fear, depression, anger, pleasure, laughter, crying
Visual, Auditory, Olfactory	Illusions and Hallucinations

Diagnosis Testing
Medical history - family, trauma, infection, toxic exposure
Laboratory Testing - serum glucose, CBC, chem screen
Imaging - CT scan, MRI, EEG

Differential Diagnosis:
Medical Disorders:
Seizure Disorders, Cerebrovascular Accident (CVA), Myocardial Infarction, Transient Ischemic Attack (TIA)
Effects of Substances:
Alcohol or illicit substance intoxication or withdrawal, Side effects of medications
Psychiatric Disorders:
Conversion Disorder, anxiety disorders, disorders of impulse control, Borderline Personality Disorder (BPD), Histrionic Personality Disorder (HPD), Schizophrenia and other psychotic disorders, Major depressive episode, Pseudoseizures

Factors Influencing the Decision to Treat
-Abnormal EEG
-Previous seizure
-Driver
-Other neurological impairment
-Elderly

Factors Influencing the Decision Not to Treat
-Single seizure
-No history
-Neurologically normal
-Young age
-Side effects

Potential Contributing Factors
Aspartic Acid Excess
Asparagine Excess
Taurine Deficiency

Contraindicator of
Aspartic Acid
Asparagine

Biomedical Approaches:

Vagus Nerve Stimulation
Vagus nerve stimulation therapy is another form of treatment that may be tried when medications fail to stop seizures. The therapy is designed to prevent seizures by sending regular small pulses of electrical energy to the brain through the vagus nerve.

Surgery
When antiepileptic drugs fail to control or substantially reduce seizures, surgery on the brain may be considered. Most surgical patients are adults who have fought long and unsuccessful battles for seizure control. However, children with severe seizures are also being treated with surgery.

Ketogenic Diet
A ketogenic diet is used when drug therapy fails to adequately control seizures. This forces a child's body to burn fat continuously throughout the day. 80% of calories are derived from fat, while the rest comes from carbohydrates and protein. The amounts of food and liquid at each meal must be carefully worked out and weighed for each person. Doctors don't know precisely why a diet that mimics starvation by burning fat for energy should prevent seizures, although this is being studied. Nor is it known why the same diet works for some children and not for others. Attempting such a diet on a child without medical guidance puts a child at risk of serious consequences. Every step of the ketogenic diet process must be managed by an experienced treatment team, usually based at a specialized medical center.

A child on the diet usually continues to take anti-seizure medicine, but may be able to take less of it later on. If a child does very well, the doctor may slowly taper the medication with the goal of discontinuing it altogether. About a third of children who try the ketogenic diet become seizure free, or nearly seizure free. Another third improve but still have some seizures. The rest either do not respond at all or find it too hard to continue with the diet, either because of side effects or because they can't tolerate the food.

Natural Treatment Approaches

Lifestyle Considerations
-Regulate sleep patterns and have a regular, consistent sleep schedule
-Identify and eliminate any environmental toxin exposure (heavy metals, chemicals)
-Identify and eliminate any food allergies

Dietary Considerations
-Food complements: kelp. Take 4-5g. of seaweed at mealtime once a day (powder in capsules or tablets)

Orthomolecular Considerations
-Glucosamine: may dampen brain hyperexcitability[1]
-Taurine
-Essential fatty acids
-Vitamin B1
-Vitamin B6 (50mg TID)
-Vitamin D
-Vitamin E (400 IU)
-Folic Acid (.4-4mg)
-Magnesium (10mg TID)
-Manganese (10mg TID)
-Zinc (25mg)
-Selenium
-Cholne
-Alanine
-GABA
-Melatonin

Acupressure/Tapping Considerations
KI-1, GV-26, GV-16, GB-20, Ear Shenmen

Research Studies:
- Electroacupuncture was tested to determine the effects of low-frequency (10 Hz) simulation of acupoint GB-20 (Fengchi) on epilepsy. Electroencephalogram (EEG) results showed that electroacupuncture significantly suppresses brain epileptiform discharges and simultaneously improves sleep patterns. The researchers note that low frequency stimulation of GB-20 suppresses epilepsy and "blocks sleep disruption". The investigators cite research showing that opioid peptides and their receptors mediate the therapeutic effects of acupuncture. Han et al. demonstrate that 2 Hz electroacupuncture stimulates an increase of met-enkephalin but not dynorphin. However, 100 Hz electroacupuncture increases dynorphin release and not met-enkephalin. [2,3]

- 60 patients with epilepsy were randomly divided into a control group and an acupuncture group. The control group received only the pharmaceutical medication sodium valproate. The acupuncture group received both scalp acupuncture and body acupuncture plus sodium valproate. The acupuncture group demonstrated significantly superior patient outcomes over the medication only group.
Scalp Acupuncture: Chest Area, Epilepsy-control area, chorea-tremor ares.
Body Acupuncture: GB-20, GV-20, Si Shen Cong, Yintang, GV-26, PC-6, LI-4, ST-36, ST-40, SP-6, LR-3.
A total of 10 days comprised one course of care. There was a 2 day break following each course of care. The treatment period was 3 months. After completion 12 acupuncture patients showed no epilepsy related symptoms for at least 1 year. A total of 9 patients showed excellent improvements and 6 patients showed moderate improvements. The overall effective rate for the acupuncture group was 90.00% compared with 73.33% for the medication control group. The researchers concludes that acupuncture combined with sodium valproate has a synergistic clinical effect leading to improved patient outcomes.[4]

- Auricular acupuncture and body style electroacupuncture reduced neuron overexcitation while simultaneously stopping epileptic seizures. Acupuncture's ability to regulate the

TRPA1 ion (active in acute pain and neurogenic inflammation) signaling channel located on the plasma membrane of cells was quantified. Auricular and electroacupuncture demonstrate the ability to halt inflammation related to epileptic seizures while simultaneously downregulating TRPA1 in the hippocampus. The auricular acupuncture group received 2 Hz electroacupuncture stimulation from the ear apex to the ear lobe for 20 minutes on the left ear and 10 minutes on the right ear per session. The body style electroacupuncture group received 2 Hz electroacupuncture from acupoints ST-36 to ST-37. Both groups were treated 3 days per week for a total of 6 weeks. Ear and body acupuncture were effective in providing relief from epileptic seizures and both types of acupuncture regulated the TRPA1 signaling pathway and additional signaling pathways: PKC, pERK1/2.

5

Chapter 16
Chronic Pain

The most common pain condition following a brain injury tend to be headaches, a topic specifically talked about in chapter 9. This chapter will focus on other forms of body pain that can often develop. Some more common conditions that are reported include head/neck pain, back pain, complex regional pain syndrome (CRPS), and fibromyalgia; among others. Pain can be due to tissue damage, spasticity or contracture, falls, etc. Service members run the additional risk of exposure to blast injuries with possible burns, traumatic amputation, high temperature gas inhalation and physical displacement injuries. In order for pain to be considered "chronic" it must have had lasted for 6 months.

There is an increasing amount of evidence showing that in chronic post-injury pain, persistent pain can be associated with what is referred to as "central sensitization". This is where the pain relay system becomes more responsive over time or will spontaneously discharge without direct stimulation causing random acute pain. This sensitization has been associated with dysfunctional functioning of the anterior cingulate cortex.

Post-traumatic stress situations have also shown to be more prone to the development of chronic pain. In some there has not been any actual physical trauma at all; rather the onset, maintenance, severity and exacerbation of pain is associated with psychological factors. Even with physical trauma present, stressors can worsen pain conditions. In cases of brain injury it has been found that complaints of pain conditions were more than twice as frequent in those who sustained a mild brain trauma compared to a more severe injury. By the same token, chronic pain can impair or worsen cognitive functioning. This is particularly true with attention, processing speed, memory, and executive functions. Chronic pain has been further associated with mood change or emotional distress, pain "catastrophization", sleep disturbance, fatigue, and chronic stress due to interference of daily activities.

The neuroanatomy of pain is a complex system that is still not completely understood. Nociceptive receptors are found in the skin, muscular and organ structures of the body. Chronic pain has been associated with a decreased density of the prefrontal and thalamic grey matter, as well as stress-induced hypothalamic-pituitary-axis dysfunction, serotonin deficiency, and increased norepinephrine levels.

Pain may also be distinguished as affecting either the lateral or medial pain systems. While there is a significant overlap between the two systems (which creates a unitary experience of pain in the individual) the following distinctions can be made:

Lateral Pain System	Medial Pain System
-Primarily sensory-discriminatory components of pain -Associated more with acute pain -Inputs to thalamus and somatosensory cortex	-Primarily emotional-motivational components of pain -Associated more closely with chronic pain- Projections of medial-thalamic nuclei to the anterior cingulate and forebrain -Sensitization with limbic structures seem to mediate pain response

Brain Regions and Pain:
Subcortical injuries (especially of the thalamus, less often with the anterior cingulate) can cause sensation loss or an inability to react to pain. At the neocortical level, while pain responsiveness may be diminished or absent after tissue damage, simple sensation remains and the ability to differentiate is retained. For example, someone can still differentiate between dull and sharp. This deficit usually affects both sides.

Cortical Region	Role in Sensation
Somatosensory Areas 1 & 2	Pain, touch, temperature sense, pressure sense, position sense, vibration sense, sensation of movement
Prefrontal area	Pain, executive function, creativity, planning, empathy, action, emotional balance, intuition
Anterior Cingulate	Pain, emotional self-control, sympathetic control, conflict detection, problem solving
Posterior Parietal Lobe	Pain, sensory, visual, auditory perception, mirror neurons, internal location of stimuli, location of external space
Supplementary Motor Zone	Pain, planned movement, mirror neurons
Amygdala	Pain, emotion, emotional memory, emotional response, pleasure, sight, smell, emotional extremes
Insula	Pain, quiets the amygdala, temperature, itch, empathy, emotional self-awareness, sensual touch, connects emotion with bodily sensation, mirror neurons, disgust
Posterior Cingulate	Pain, visuospatial cognition, autobiographical memory retrieval
Hippocampus	Helps to store pain memories
Orbital Frontal Cortex	Pain, evaluates whether something is pleasant vs. unpleasant, empathy, understanding, emotional attunement

Diagnostic Assessment
-Self-report
     -Visual Analog Scale (rate severity 1-10)
     -Numerical Analogue Scale
     -Onset, pallative, quality, radiation, severity, timing
     -Intake of pre-injury pain levels, pain vulnerabilities, relevant family history, etc.
-Psychological assessment
-Nociception Coma Scale (for those with disorders of consciousness)

Biomedical Approach

Treatment Approaches for Pain		
Analgesics	Antidepressants	Anticonvulsants
-Acetaminophen -Tramadol -Steroids -Prednisone -Dexamethasone	-Amitriptyline -Desipramine -Nortriptyline -Fluoxetine -Paroxetine -Duloxetine	-Carbamazepine -Valproic Acid -Phenytoin -Clonazepam -Gabapentin -Levetiracetam -Lamotrigine -Oxcarbazepine -Pregabalin
Opioids	Local Anesthetics	Topical Anesthetics
-Morphine -Hydromorphone -Codeine -Hydrocordone -Oxycodone -Meperidine -Fentanyl	-Lidocaine -Mexiletine -Flecainide	-Capsaicin -"Speed Gel"
Physical Modalities	Behavioral Treatments	
-Hot/cold Packs -Heat Lamps -Parrafin baths -Laser therapy -Cryotherpay -Hydrotherapy -Ultrasound -Phonopheresis -Diathermy Transcutaneous nerve stimulations (TENS) -Iontophoresis -Cranial electrotherapy stimulation (CES) -Traction -Injections – prolotherapy, trigger point, plasma -Epidural -Sympathetic blocks -Vestibular stimulation	-Patient education -Biofeedback -Relaxation training -Operant treatment -Cognitive-behavioral treatment -Social and assertive skills training -Imagery -Hypnosis -Habit Reversal -Body mechanics and ergonomics training	

Natural Treatment Approaches

Lifestyle Considerations
-Meditation/mindfulness
-Group counseling/pain support groups
-Individual counseling/pain management therapy

Body Based Considerations
-Topical liniments
-Exercise/stretching affected area

Dietary Considerations
-Mediterranean Diet
-Anti-inflammatory foods
-Avoid: inflammatory foods and foods sensitivities

Orthomolecular Considerations
-Bromelain
-Gaba-linoleic acid
-Vitamin C
-Vitamin D
-SAMe
-Omega 3 Fatty Acids
-Probiotics

Phytotherapeutic Considerations

-Turmeric/Curcumin   -Clove Oil
-Capsaicin   -Ginger
-Arnica   -Fennel
-Boswellia   -Feverfew
-Willow Bark   -Green Tea
-Devil's Claw   -Licorice Root

Acupressure/Tapping Considerations

Point Recommendations Based on Pain Location₁	
Upper Extremities	Lower Extremities
PC-6	KI-1
LI-11	LR-4
ST-12	SP-6
LU-9	KI-6
CV-17	GB-34

Chapter 17
Neuralgia and Numbness

Neuralgia is a pain that follows the path of a specific nerve tract. The causes of neuralgia can vary greatly. Trauma, chemical irritation, inflammation, compression of nerves by nearby structures like tight muscles, and infections may all lead to neuralgia.

Trigeminal neuralgia is the most common form of neuralgia and is a result of inflammation or compression of the trigeminal nerve which runs along the side of the face. A related but rather uncommon neuralgia affects the glossopharyngeal nerve, which provides sensation to the throat. Symptoms of this neuralgia are short, shock-like episodes of pain located in the throat. The occipital nerve can also be affected, causing occipital neuralgia in the back of the neck and scalp. Partial or full paralysis or loss of sensation can also occur along a nerve trajectory.

Neurogenic pain or discomfort may actually increase temporarily as feeling and/or range of motion increases with treatment. This feels similar to a body part that has "fallen asleep" with discomfort as it "wakes up" until full neural signaling is reestablished. This can be uncomfortable and it is important to keep in mind this is temporary.

Biomedical Approaches
-Gabapentin (Neurontin)
-SSRI's
        -Fluoxetine (Prozac)
        -Citalopram (Celexa)
        -Paroxetime (Paxil)
        -Bupropion (Wellbutrin)
Sedatives
        -Clonazepam (Klonopin)
Anticonvulsants
        -Carbamazepine (Tegretol)
        -Oxcarbazepine (Trileptal
        -Lamotrigine (Lamictal)
        -Phentoin (Dilantin)
-Anti-spasmotics
        -Baclofen (Gablofen)
-Botox injections
-Glycerol injections
-Microvascular decompression surgery
-Nerve blocks
-Nerve ablation

Differential Diagnosis
-Diabetic neuropathy
-Nerve compression
-Herpes Zoster (Shingles)
-Post-herpetic neuralgia

-Renal insufficiency
-Polyphyria
-Drug use

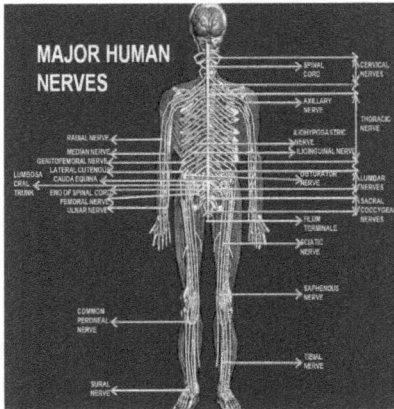

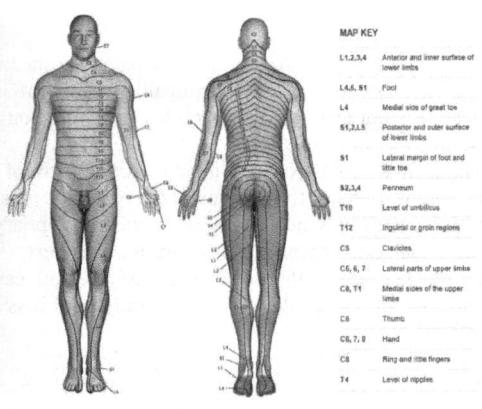

Natural Treatment Approaches

Dietary Considerations
Eat food which contains a good source of vitamin B1, such as yeast, wheat germ, egg yolks, carrots, whole wheat bread, parsley, spinach, and rosemary.

Orthomolecualr Considerations
-Magnesium
-Vitamin C
-Vitamins B1 (thiamine), B6, B9 (folic acid), B12
-Vitamin D
-Vitamin E
-Biotin
-5-HTP
-GABA
-Omega 6 fatty acids
-CoQ10
-**Alpha lipoic acid**
-Acetyl L-Carnitine
-N-Acetylcysteine (NAC)
-L-Glutamine
-Taurine

Phytotherapeutic Considerations
-Angelica
-Capsaicin
-Cayenne
-Curcumin/Turmeric
-Kava kava

138

-Evening Primrose Oil
-Skullcap
-Feverfew
-Oats
-Colloidal Silver

Body-based Considerations
-Regular massage
-Liniments (Zheng Gu Shui, liquid magnesium, etc.)
-Herbal Compresses
-Plum Blossom along affected nerve tract(s)

Acupressure/Tapping Considerations

Point Recommendations Based on Pain Location[1]	
Upper Extremities	Lower Extremities
PC-6	KI-1
LI-11	LR-4
ST-12	SP-6
LU-9	KI-6
CV-17	GB-34

Chapter 18
Movement Disorders and Paralysis

Movement disorders that develop following an injury can either be transient or persistent. They are estimated to be present in between 13-66% of TBI survivors. One of the largest studies showed persistent symptoms in 12.2 % with the most common forms being tremor and dystonia (muscle spasms and unnatural posture). Many people have to completely relearn to walk or to use a limb after an injury. Younger people tend to show a greater tendency toward generalized muscle dystonia. Movement disorders are generally placed into the following categories:

-Hyperkinetic disorders: tremor, dystonia, ballism (jerking or flinching)
-Tics, Chorea (unpredictable dance-like movements)
-Tourettism (Semi-voluntary repetative movements or vocalizations)
-Sudden shock-like movements, cramps (myoclonus)
-Exaggerated startle response (hyperekplexia)
-Sense of inner restlessness (akathisia)
-Hypokinetic disorders: Parkinsonism, rigidity, resting tremor, postural instability

Paralyis and muscular atrophy can develop as a result of direct parietal lobe damage of the sensorimotor cortex. Lesions or tumors to the right lobe seem to be particularly impactful, affecting the associated region of the opposite side of the body. If there is a loss of sensation, an individual may lose a sense of their body within space, which in turn can generate motor disturbances such as paresis with reduced muscle tone or a reduction in the ability ("will") to initiate movement. Peripheral nerve injuries that no longer allow for full conduction of nerve impulses to the appendages, as well as progressive inflammation and cytotoxicity from diffuse axonal injury, may also cause paralysis. Single-sided spasticity (hemiplegia) of a limb or side of the body can frequently occur when the appropriate brain regions are affected. Ataxia, a condition where there is a loss of full control of one's bodily movements can also occur and be difficult to treat.

Biomedical Approaches
-Baclofen (spasticity)
-Beta-blockers (ataxia)
-Stereotactic surgery (ataxia)

Natural Treatment Approaches

Dietary Considerations
-Foods which help nourish the Blood and Sinews

Orthomoelcular Considerations
-Magnesium (oral or topical)
-L-Dopa

Phytotherapeutic Considerations
-Bai Shao Gan Cao Wan, a simple two herb formula consisting of licorice root and white

peony root can be added to other herbal prescriptions or as a standalone prescription in cases of spasticity, contracture and paralysis

Somatic Considerations
-Sotai
-Positional Release Techniques
-Massage
-Qigong
-Tai Ji Quan
-Moxa
-Plum Blossom
-Cold laser/Tens stimulation

-Often Japanese Sotai techniques can be used as a gentle movement modality to assist in range of motion improvement in cases where muscles and tendons spasticity or contracture is present

Movement Exercise Considerations
-Theraband resistance and assistance
-Calf raises
-Stress ball, finger strengthening tools (hands)
-Playing an instrument (hands/fingers)
-Foot peddle (feet/ankle)
-Tracing out the alphabet with your hands and/or feet

Acupressure/Tapping Considerations
LI-4, LI-10, LI-11, ST-36, ST-41, GB-34, GB-41, TW-5

Chapter 19
Hormonal Dysregulation

It has been recorded that up to two thirds of individuals who sustain a brain injury experience single or multiple pituitary-target hormone disruptions. 20% of those affected have a combination of two or more deficiencies, many being transient in nature. Hypopituitarism is considered a common sequela of brain injury and it has been suggested that pituitary cells are particularly vulnerable to trauma. This dysregulation more commonly affects the gonadal or growth hormone (15%) channels of the endocrine system, though a wide array of channels and regulatory functions can be affected.

Common Endocrine Disturbances Following a Brain Injury	
-Hypo/hyperthyroidism	-Hyperprolactinemia
-Impaired growth hormone release	-Temperature dysregulation
-Impaired adrenal cortical function	-Inappropriate diuretic hormone syndrome
-Hypopituitarism	-Diabetes insipidus
-Hypothalamic hypogonadism	-Menstrual irregularities
-Precocious puberty	-Changes in sexual function
-Hyperphagia	

Some of these concerns will be specifically addressed in following chapters. The mechanisms of these effects has been identified as the result of a direct mechanical injury, cytotoxic processes, or both. This occurs to the central nervous system components of the hypothalamic-pituitary-organ axes. Injury of the pituitary lobe can also result from compression or occlusion of the surrounding blood vessels stemming from brain swelling and edema.

Thyroid Dysfunction - Hypothyroidism
Diagnosis
myxedema
thyroid hormone deficiency

Etiology
primary
Autoimmune
-Hashimoto's thyroiditis
-Chronic influence of thyroid with lymphocytic infiltration caused by autoimmune factors
-8:1 more in women
-Often family history of thyroid disorders

post-therapeutic
-Surgery
-Drugs for hyperthyroidism

-Iodine deficiency - goiter

secondary
- Decrease in thyroid stimulating hormone from hypothalamus
- Decrease in thyroid stimulating hormone from pituitary

Signs & Symptoms of Hypothyroidism		
- Insidious onset - Fatigue - Dull facies with periorbital edema - Hoarse voice, slow speech - Cold intolerance, hypothermia - Coarse, dry, thin hair - Coarse, dry, scaly, thick skin - Weight gain	- Memory and intellectual impairment - Constipation - Paresthesias - Brisk contraction, slow relaxation of reflexes - Macroglossia - Bradycardia - Pericardial, pleural effusion	- Carotenodermia (orange skin on palms and soles) - Menorrhagia - Anemia - Thyroid may be enlarged, tender or non-tender, smooth or nodular, firm or rubbery - **if nodular, refer for evaluation**

Diagnostic Testing
1. decreased serum T4 (thyroxine) [normal: 0.5-5.0, some suggest higher than 2.5 is troublesome]
2. decreased T3 uptake (triiodothyronine)
3. elevated or decreased TSH (thyroid stimulating hormone)

Biomedical Approaches

- Replacement therapy : desiccated thyroid [contains T1, T2, T3, T4], L-thyroxine (synthroid, levoxyl) [only T4]
- Iodine 4 mg/d
- Vitamin D helps T3 bind to receptors
-Tyrosin

Natural Treatment Approaches

-Armour thyroid hormone
-Hydrotherapy (cold)
-Exercise – stimulate thyroid production
-Physical therapy

Orthomolecular Considerations
-Zinc (25mg)
-Selenium
-Vitamin B2
-Copper (5mg)

-Antioxidants (vitamin C, vitamin E, turmeric)

Thyroid Dysfunction - Hyperthyroidism
thyrotoxicosis - Grave's Disease

Etiology
- Unknown, but probably immunologic

Signs and Symptoms of Hyperthyroidism	
- Nervousness, increased activity	**in Grave's disease**
- Increased perspiration, heat intolerance	- Exophthalmos
- Fatigue, weakness	- Ocular muscle weakness
- Increased appetite, weight loss	- Pretibial edema
- Insomnia	- Non-pitting, pruritic edema
- Frequent bowel movements	
- Goiter	
- Tachycardia, atrial fibrillation	
- Warm, moist skin	
- Tremor	
- Stare	

Diagnostic Testing
- Decreased TSH
- Elevated free T4
- Elevated T3 uptake
- Elevated T3

Biomedical Treatment
- Anti-thyroid agents – Propylthiouracil, Methimazole (Tapazole)
- Radioactive iodine
- Surgery

Chapter 20
Incontinence and Bowel Disorders

Due to the brain housing the regulatory system for bowel and bladder function, a brain injury can disturb control over these functions and result in urinary or fecal incontinence.

Urinary Incontinence
Urinary incontinence tends to be associated with bilateral central injuries. Someone will often experience an altered bladder sensation, lowered capacity, increased sense of urgency and greater frequency. Damage to the spinal cord or sacral nerve roots can also cause urinary incontinence. Urinary tract infections (UTI) can happen both early after injury and long after the initial incident.

Approaches to urinary incontinence include
-Maintaining adequate hydration
-Minimizing intake of caffeine and caramel colored drinks
-Timed voiding
-Use of cranberry tablets or D-Mannose
-Early detection and treatment of UTI.

If incontinence persists even after time-voiding training there may be a bladder study performed and a referral to a urologist familiar with brain injury related bladder concerns. The urologist may recommend medications, generally anti-cholinergics, an external portable collection device, or adult disposable briefs may be considered.

Fecal Incontinence
Fecal incontinence does not occur as frequently, though it has been associated with similar brain and spinal pathways to those that regulate bladder function. Diarrhea, constipation, impaction, or bowel obstruction may result from changes in mobility, tube feedings, food consistency, intake status, fluid intake and medication. The impact of narcotics on bowel regularity, as used for acute and chronic pain management, is a challenge for many and is of particular concern. Good bowel hygiene, including a routine that promotes emptying at least two or three times weekly, are necessary for the establishment of bowel continence and regularity. Ensuring dietary and fluid intakes include enough bulk, roughage and fluid to aid in regularity. Medications used to restore and maintain bowel emptying including stool softeners, irritant cathartics that promote bowel regularity, bulk laxatives, suppositories or low volume enemas may be used.

Individuals should be assessed for signs of constipation or impaction including abdominal distention, nausea and decreased appetite. Other signs of autonomic dysregulation such as high blood pressure and sweating may also indicate impaction. While constipation itself is not a critical disorder, the complications that can accompany constipation certainly can be. Continued constipation can result in an auto-intoxication due to resorption of toxins in the intestines. Symptoms of auto intoxication include dizziness, headache, loss of appetite, irritability, insomnia, acne, and dry, cracking or peeling skin. Chronic constipation can also lead to stubborn disorders including hemorrhoids, fissures and fistulas, and abscesses. It can also provoke a medical crisis like a heart attack due to forcing and straining during defecation.

If cognitive functioning is affected, the brain injured individual may be a poor reporter of bowel emptying which can be an issue for caregivers.

Brain Injury in Conjunction with Spinal Cord Injury
If someone has both a brain injury and spinal cord injury they may not be able to feel or control their bowels. When this is the case, proper and routine bowel care become necessary to prevent further complications such as constipation or auto-intoxication. This consists of a bowel program as well as assistance for the individual in eating properly: a high fiber diet, drinking adequate fluids to ensure proper hydration and being active through exercise. In cases where the individual requires a wheelchair this means getting up from the chair at regular intervals.

Bladder control is also a concern here. Kidney disease was recently the leading cause of death in individuals with spinal cord injury. Necessary focus includes preventing UTI, maintaining low pressure urine storage, and (if able) voiding without urinary leakage or over-distention of the urinary bladder. Management usually entails an indwelling catheter, an intermittent catheter, or in cases of men with a reflexic bladder, an external collector. Intermittent cathetization has a reduced risk of infection and is generally preferred despite associated risks of urethral trauma and blood in the urine. An individual with memory problems may have difficulty remembering to maintain the 4-6 hour schedule of an intermittent catheter.

Natural Treatment Approaches

-Stress incontinence can be treated with regular Kegel exercises outlined below. These exercises help strengthen the muscles that control the bladder and can be done anywhere, at any time. It may take 3 to 6 months to see an improvement so patients must be persistent and patient.

Kegel exercises
-To locate the right muscles, try stopping or slowing your urine flow without using your stomach, leg or buttock muscles. When you're able to slow or stop the stream of urine, you've located the right muscles.
- Squeeze your muscles. Hold for a count of 10. Relax for a count of 10.
- Repeat this 10 to 20 times, 3 times a day.
- You may need to start slower, perhaps squeezing and relaxing your muscles for 4 seconds each and doing this 10 times, 2 times a day. Work your way up from there.

Bladder training for urge incontinence:
Some people who have urge incontinence can learn to lengthen the time between urges to go to the bathroom. Start by urinating at set intervals, such as every 30 minutes to 2 hours (whether you feel the need to go or not). Then gradually lengthen the time between urinating (for example, by 30 minutes) until it is every 3 to 4 hours. Relaxation techniques can be practiced when the urge to urinate is felt before it is time to go to the bathroom.

148

Breathe slowly and deeply.

Think about the breath until the urge goes away. Kegel exercises can also be done if they help control urgency. After the urge passes, wait 5 minutes and then go to the bathroom even if there is no feeling of needing to urinate. When it's easy to wait 5 minutes after an urge, begin waiting 10 minutes. Bladder training may take 3 to 12 weeks.

Bowel Incontinence

Etiology
Osmotic: non-absorbable, water-soluble solutes in bowel - lactose, simple carbohydrates
Secretory: secrete electrolytes and water - bacterial toxins, viruses
Exudative: mucosal inflammation and ulceration
Decreased intestinal transit time: not enough exposure to absorptive surface for a sufficient amount of time - 18-30hrs. is pretty average

Potential Contributing Factors
-Dysbiosis
-Magnesium Excess
-Potassium Excess

Potential Secondary Effects
-Excess blood potassium (Hypokalaemia)

Parasitic infections
- Entameba histolytica
- Giardia lamblia
- Enterobius vermicularis [pinworm]
- Diagnosis by Ovum & Parasite exam

Biomedical Approaches
- Find and treat underlying disorder
- Rehydration (water alone is not best - electrolytes, etc.)
- Avoid simple carbohydrates
- Charcoal
- Rice water
- Psyllium seed (Fiberall, Metamucil)
- Difenoxin (Motofen)
- Diphenoxylate (Lomotil, Lonox)
- Acidophilus
- Hydrastis (Goldenseal)

10-12 bowel movements a day may be an infection of candida

Clinical Notes:
-With proper treatment, most cases of diarrhea resolve in a few days; however, inappropriate treatment can prolong recovery and lead to chronic diarrhea. Pathological crisis related to diarrhea is rare. Severe, excessive and unremitting diarrhea, however, will lead to severe loss of body fluids. Clinical manifestations of this type of crisis include

149

intense thirst with desire to drink, profuse leading and cold extremities, pale complexion and minute pulse. Biomedically, this is termed a fluid and electrolyte imbalance.

Natural Treatment Approaches

Dietary Considerations
-Remove all simple carbohydrates

Orthomolecular Considerations
-Sodium
-Potassium
-Charcoal
-Chlorine (persistant)
-Active Lactobaccillus

Phytotherapeutic Considerations
-Vinca Minor (Periwinkle)

Acupressure/Tapping Considerations
ST-36, LI-4, LI-11, CV-6, CV-12, ST-25

Constipation

Signs & Symptoms
- 3-5 stools per week
- More than 3 days without stool
- Stool weight less than 35gm

Etiology
- Obstruction
- Drugs
- Tumors
- Functional disorders
- IBS, hypothyroidism
- Psychological

Potential Contributing Factors
-Variations in blood calcium levels
-Arginine Deficiency

Complications
-Hemorrhoids
-Diverticulosis
-Colon Cancer

Biomedical Approaches
-Hydration, fiber, allergies, exercise
-Psyllium (Fiberall, Metamucil)
-Laculose (Constulose, Enulose, Generlac, Kristalose)
-Polyethylene Glycol (Colyte, GoLYTELY, Gycolax, Miralax, NuLYTELY, Trylite)
- Abdominal massage
- Magnesium, vitamin C

Natural Treatment Approaches

-Abdominal massage can help to regulate or initiate peristalsis
-Consider allergies, particularly milk, if there is alternating constipation/diarrhea

Dietary Recommendations
- Drink 2 liters of water/day.
- Eat vegetable fibers which are necessary for a healthy intestinal tract: green vegetables and fruit, bran (cholesterol must be lowered), muscilages.
- Avoid spicy food.
- Eat whole wheat organic bread (bran), cooked prunes, prune juice, green vegetables, fresh figs.
- No pulses or bananas
- Psyllium powder

Orthomolecular Treatment
- Magnesium 600-900 mg/day
- Vitamin C 10gms/day
- Glucomannan
- Fructo-oligosaccharides
- Vitamin B complex

Acupressure/Tapping Considerations
ST-36, ST-37, LI-11, CV-4, CV-12, ST-25

Research Studies
1. In a controlled investigation, acupuncture plus topical herbal medicine had a higher total effective rate and a higher complete recovery rate than drug therapy for post-stroke constipation. In addition, acupuncture plus topical herbal medicine had a significantly lower failure rate than drug therapy. [1]

Chapter 21
Sexual Dysfunction

Given that the brain is involved in all aspects of hormonal regulation and sexual functioning; a brain injury can result in changes in libido, arousal and sexual performance. This includes everything from stimulus, ability to communicate in forming intimate relationships, awareness of excitement, to the physiological responses that happen at cognitive, neurological, and genital levels. Sexuality involves multiple brain regions including the frontal lobes, limbic structures and the temporal lobes. Injuries to the right hemisphere are particularly important. These changes in sexuality can be further compounded by hormonal changes and medication side-effects.

Trauma to the pituitary gland can disrupt hormonal levels in the body which can cause disruption of menstrual cycles in women or affect testosterone levels. Reproductive health can become a prominent concern as UTI's, painful periods, polycystic ovarian symptoms, and pre-menstrual mood dysphoria become possible along with accompanying depression, hormonally regulated migraines, osteoporosis or endocrine disorders.

Women with a TBI may be limited in their use of oral contraceptives or estrogen replacement therapy as a result of deep vein thrombosis (DVT) or embolus post-injury. Medications can cause menopause to come on earlier. This is particularly true of anti-seizure medications. Seizures on the hypothalamic-pituitary axis can worsen this situation.

Hygiene can also become a concern for some affected by a brain injury who may not be able to fully tend to their own hygiene. Routine gynecological, testicular, and prostate examinations, contraceptive counseling, awareness of STD risk should be given consideration for individuals.

Hormonal treatment of progesterone or estrogen have been studied as an acute injury treatment approach. Progesterone modulates GABA and inhibits cell death and the production of inflammatory agents. Estrogen is a powerful antioxidant which also protects the blood vessels. In animal models estrogen treatment seemed to only show benefit for males, while females showed the treatment to be detrimental and with increased injury-related mortality risk.

Possible Effects on Sexuality
The American Brain Injury Association cites 10 notable areas in which sexuality may be affected by a brain injury:

Difficulty with Sexual Energy, Desire or Drive
This may be because of general fatigue following a brain injury or one's ability to manage sleep, stress and health habits. Some find that they have less interest in all life drives, including sexual. This may cause difficulty in maintaining romantic relationships despite being a neurobiological issue, not one reflecting the feelings felt for another, the value placed on the relationship, or the perceived attractiveness by the individual.

Reduction/Loss of Sensation or Orgasm

An injury can effect the neural circuitry that carries signals of feeling pleasure that lead to orgasm. Additionally, many prescription medications can have this same effect.

Positioning, Movement, and Pain Difficulties
Due to pain or difficulties in movement following an injury, certain movements or sexual positions can be limited. These may be addressed through physical therapy, physiotherapies that reduce pain, and the possible use of adaptive positioning aids.

Altered Body Image, Mood, and Self-Confidence
Depression, a loss of confidence, or reduced self-esteem has been associated with brain injury in up to 50% of cases for both men and women. This may additionally stem from, or be compounded by, disability, unemployment, or changes in family or social roles.

Decreased Ability To Sexually Satisfy One's Partner
Individuals may not be able to remember the proper exchanges or patterns of interaction involved in intimacy. Due to increased mental and physical expenditure, someone may not be able to process these exchanges in the moment. When interacting with a partner after an injury both parties may have to be patient in relearning one another. Couples counseling may be helpful in order to effectively communicate with one another and reestablish new foundations between them.

Disinhibition and Hypersexuality
Hypersexuality does not seem to occur as frequently as disinterest, however it can cause a number of issues for those affected. In cases where the frontal lobe has been injured it is possible that the inhibitory function on the base animalistic drives of the limbic system and lower brain centers may fail. This can result in uninhibited offensive comments, changes in character behaviors, and seemingly, a loss of moral judgment and ability to gauge social appropriateness. This may include compulsive sexual pursuit, exhibitionism, touching themselves or others in public, lack of regard for rights or space of others, and little regard for cultural norms, situational contexts, religious teachings or traditions. The individual may proposition caregivers, strangers, friends or family. They may patronize prostitutes and there is the possibility of developing violent sexual behavior that was unknown prior to injury. This can cause difficulty for the individual or among family members, caretakers or medical practitioners. Severe cases may require inpatient care.

Incontinence and Issues of Adaptive Equipment
An individual who experiences bowel or bladder incontinence may avoid sexual activity due to embarrassment of these issues or out of fear of an accident. Management of a voiding schedule may assist in this matter and may be addressed with their healthcare provider.

Diminished Capacity for Sexual Ideation
One's ability to think about or imagine sexual activity can be affected. This may further reduce one's drive and interest in sexual matters. Counseling and increased communication among partners may assist in this matter.

Greater Sexual Concerns Among Those With Mild TBI
An injury that is mild may recover quite well but have persistent symptoms. Because the individual is more consciously aware of any deficits or difficulties than those with severe brain injury, this can be of great concern and may exacerbate depression.

Sexual Intimacy Issues May Predate TBI
It is important to be aware of any intimacy concerns present prior to the onset of injury.

Primary Causes of Sexual Dysfunction	
-Neuroendocrine/hormonal changes	-Hypothalamus and Pituitary Damage: 40-62% of persons have shown pituitary damage, 42% showed hypothalamic lesions

Secondary Causes of Sexual Dysfunction	
Physical Changes	Cognitive Impairments
-Spasticity -Hemiparesis -Ataxia -Balance -Movement disorders -Sensory deficits	-Attention and Concentration -Initiation (motivation to act) -Social Communication Abilities -Impaired Awareness -Memory Loss -Executive Dysfunction
Emotional and Behavioral Changes	Other Potential Factors
-Depression -Child-like or Dependency Behaviors -Self-centeredness -Apathy/Decreased Initiation -Disinhibition or Trouble Self-monitoring -Low Self-Esteem or Poor Body Image	-Marital or Family Dysfunction -Role Changes -Financial Stress -Parenting Strain -Decreased Communication Between Partners -Social Isolation -Medication Side Effects

Effects of Certain Medication Classes on Sexual Functioning			
Drug Category	Examples	Potential Benefits	Potential Effects on Sexual Functionin
Antidepressants	Prozac, Elavil, Norpramin	Control/Improves Mood	Delays Orgasm, Anorgasma (Not Wellbutrin)
Antispasmodics	Probathine, Baclofen	Reduce/Control Spasms	Modifies sensory experience of orgasm
Antipsychotics	Zyprexa, Seroquel, Haldol	Control /Improve psychotic symptoms	Decreases sexual drive, increases fatigue, delays orgasm, esp. older medications
Antihypertensives	Inderol, Beta blockers	Control blood pressure	Decreases sexual drive, erectile

155

			dysfunction
Stimulants	Ritalin, Adderal	Improve attention, enhance cognition	Increases sexual drive, decreases fatigue
Antiseizure	Dilantin, Tegretol, Depakote	Reduce/control seizures	Decreases sexual drive, increases fatigue, disinterest
Antihistamine	Actifed, Atarax, Claritin	Control Allergy Symptoms	Older medications decrease sexual drive and anorgasmic response, increase fatigue. New medications – no effects identified
Anti-inflammatory	Advil, Naprosyn	Control Inflammation and reduce pain	Increases sexual drive, decreases menstrual pain, increases sexual response
Antibiotics	Cipro, Penicillin	Control infection	May increase vaginal itching and yeast infections
Antiemetics	Reglan, Compazine	Control nausea	Decreases sexual drive, decreases orgasmic response
Oral Contraceptives	"The Pill" - various formulations	Prevents conception	Various types may either increase or decrease sexual drive
Androgen Anabolic Steroids	Winstrol, Anadrol	Minimizes wasting syndromes	Increases sexual drive, absence of menstrual period, clitoral enlargement
Hormone Replacement Therapy	Estratest, Premarin	Adjust hormone levels following menopause / hysterectomy (risk)	Increases sexual drive, prevents vaginal atrophy

Differential Diagnosis

Frontal lobe: sexual automatisms, such as "sexual hypermotoric pelvic or truncal movements" are common in frontal lobe seizures

Temporal Lobe: discrete genital automatisms, like fondling and grabbing the genitals are more common in seizures involving the temporal lobe.

In most instances, "sexual" seizures are associated with being within the right frontal lobe. However, some may also become hyposexual, especially with left frontal injuries, and/or experience genital pain with left temporal seizures.

Natural Treatment Approaches

Lifestyle Recommendations
-Increase the intake of foods with warm properties such as lamb, onions and chives.
-A balanced diet should go along with a balanced lifestyle that includes proper work hours, exercise and play
-Hypnosis (if no physiological cause)

Phytotherapeutic Considerations
-Epimedium (Yin Yang Huo)
-Cordyceps (Dong Chong Xia Cao)
-Cinnamon bark (rou Gui)

Deficiency
Low sexual response (women): Rou Cong Rong, Lu Jiao Jiao, Zi He Che, Shu Di Huang$_8$
Lack of sexual response (women): Lu Rong, Ren Shen, Shu Di, Tu Si Zi$_8$

Acupressure/Tapping Considerations
-GV-4, SP-6, CV-1, TW-5

Hypersexuality/Disinhibition

Individual herbs for sexual dysfunction
Sexual Dysfunction: Che Qian Zi, Dang Gui, Dong Chong Xia Cao, Ge Jiue, Guan Mu Tang, Hai Ma, Hai Shen, Long Gu, Ren Shen, Xiao Mao, Yin Yang Huo, Ze Xie $_9$

Excess
Sex drive increased abnormally: Zhi Mu$_8$, Bai Shao
Easily aroused: Huang Bai

Acupressure/Tapping Considerations
-HT-3, HT-8, HT-9, PC-5

Chapter 22
Visual Disturbances

Visual problems are very common following a brain injury with a number of different possible problems that may occur. Most commonly, these are concerns affecting oculomotor abnormalities, accomodative dysfunctions, dry eye, cataracts, and visual field defects. Other indirect pathologies such as orbital fractures, lid abnormalities, pupillary abnormalities, optic nerve abnormalities, and retinal defects may occur. In a sample study the most common of these included exophoric deviations (41.9%), oculomotor dysfunctions (39.7%), and visual field defects (32.5%). Vision abnormalities can negatively affect one's ability to perform daily activities such as reading, writing, walking, driving, among others.

Refractive changes may cause constant blurred vision. Reduced visual acuity can also be caused by damage along the primary visual pathway anywhere between the optic nerve head and the occipital cortex. Appropriate glasses may help adjust for these conditions.

Visual Disturbances Common in Brain Injury	
Spots (floaters)	A result of vitreous debris from degeneration of the attachment of the vitreous body to the optic nerve and retina early in life. While potentially bothersome, they do not pose much actual health risk
Retinal Detachment	Usually from trauma to the head or eye, it is typically preceded by a shower of sparks in one quadrant of the visual field, followed by a sensation like a curtain falling over the the eye
Scotomas (blind or light spot)	A negative scotoma is a blind spot in the visual field. It can often be unnoticed unless it occurs in the central vision. A positive scotoma is a light spot or scintillating flash that occurs as a response to abnormal stimulation of some portion of the visual system (e.g. during a migraine prodrome)
Myopia (nearsightedness)	The visual image strikes in front of the retina due to an elongated eyeball or excessive refractive power. The individual can see near objects but not far ones
Hyperopia (farsightedness)	The visual image strikes behind the retina due to a shortened eyeball or weak refractive power. The most common refractive error. Presbyopia is a hyperopia with advancing age as the lens hardens
Astigmatism	Refraction of the eyeball is unequal in its different meridians
Anisometropia	A different refractive error in each eye
Stabimus	Deviation of one eye. If the condition is congenital, there is no diplopia (double vision), as the vision in the deviated eye is suppressed by the brain. This suppression results in amblyopia.
Diplopia (double-vision)	This can occur for a variety of reasons.

Deficits of the Visual System		
Deficit	**Symptoms**	**Treatment Approaches**
Deficits of accommodation	Constant or intermittent blur, easy visual fatigue, inability to hold prolonged near vision, tearing, occasional headache	separate pair of reading glasses with or without vision therapy
Refractive changes	Constant blur at a particular viewing distance	Glasses
Versional ocular motility deficits	Reading difficulty, slower reading speed and loss of place when reading, texts appears to "swim", misreading or rereading words, difficulty shifting gaze or tracking objects while walking	Vision therapy Differential diagnosis: vestibular defects
Vergent ocular motility deficits	Constant or intermittent double vision, eliminated with covering one eye, easy visual fatigue, reading words may appear to "float", intermittent closing of one eye, may avoid eye contact to avoid double vision	Fusional prisms, vision therapy, Vertical oculomotor deviations: surgical intervention, visual occlusion
Visual-vestibular disturbances	Disequilibrium, dizziness with increased sensitivity to visual motion in busy environments (malls, supermarkets, etc.), accompanied by nausea and/or headache	Neurology/neurotology referral, vestibular rehabilitation (e.g. VOR training), oculomotor rehabilitation
Photosensitivity	Elevated sensitivity to light (may be selective to fluorescent lights or general)	Tinted lenses, wearing brimmed hats
Visual field impairment	Missing a portion of one's visual field with or without inattention. Having relative defects scattered throughout field of vision	Laterally displaced prism glasses, half-Fresnel prisms, mirrors

Anatomy and Visual Pathways

The eyes are more than just intimately connected to the brain, they are an actual external extension of the brain. They are the only part of the brain we are able to see. The eye is structurally made up of the cornea, conjunctiva, sclera, iris, aqeous humor, anterior and posterior chamber, crystalline lens, vitreous humor, retina, and choroid.

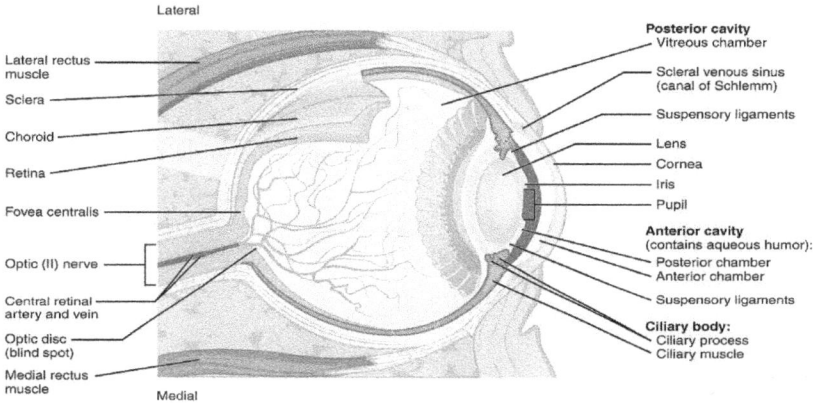

The primary visual pathway begins at the retina where two types of ganglion cell axons, magnocelluar (transient cells) and parvocelluar (sustained cells) exit as the optic nerve via the optic nerve head. These axons extend to the optic chiasm where fibers of each eye ensure visual information is kept separated to it's respective hemisphere. The visual signals then travel the optic tract to the lateral geniculate body where it is combined with non-visual neural signals. From here, fibers travel to a few different locations:
-Primary visual cortex (occipital cortex) via the optic radiations: early visual processing
-Tectum: to help pupil function
-Superior colliculus: helps in eye movement and related multisensory integrative behaviors

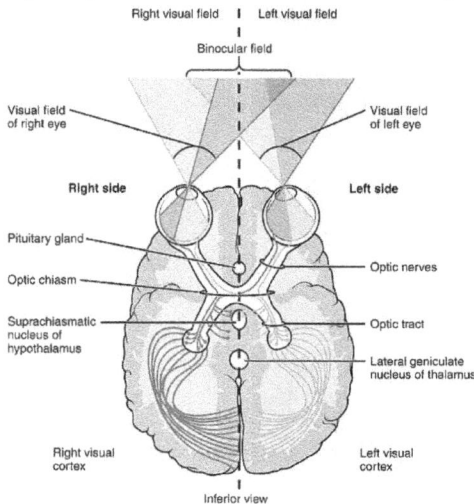

161

The secondary visual pathway begins at the visual cortex. From here the ventral visual pathway, primarily composed of parvocellular cells, is associated with visual identification and object recognition. The dorsal visual pathway, primarily composed of magnocellual cells, gauges motion and spatial vision. Other cortical areas can impact eye movement if damaged include the cerebellum, midbrain, frontal eye fields, superior colliculus, parietal cortex, and visual cortex.

Pathophysiology

Deficit	Possible Mechanism	Clinical Manifestations
Blurred Vision	Injury to cornea, lens, and/or retina Damage to the optic nerve or anywhere along the primary visual pathway Cranial nerve III damage Midbrain injury Refractive error Amblyopia Side effect of medications	Constant or intermittent blurred vision in one or both eyes Fatigue or eye strain with sustained visual tasks
Binocular Vision Abnormalities	Diminished motor control of the eye (cranial nerve 3, 4, or 6 palsy or paresis) Midbrain injury affecting medial longitudinal fasciculus and/or the oculomotor nuclei	Constant or intermittent double vision in some or all positions Depth perception inaccuracies Difficulty localizing objects in space Confusion with sustained visual activities
Nystagmus	Brainstem damage Cerebellar damage	Abnormal ocular oscillations resulting in oscillopsia, nausea, blurred vision, and visual confusion
Deficits of Pursuit	Injury in either hemisphere with or without brainstem damage	Difficulty tracking in any plane
Deficits of Saccades	Frontal eye field (area 8) and parietal injury	Difficulty in quickly locating objects Difficulty with reading

Natural Treatment Approaches
Lifestyle Considerations:
-Sufficient, regular sleep
-Ensuring proper breaks are taken during physical activity or mental work
-Regular, moderate exercise

Dietary Considerations
Therapeutic foods:
-Foods rich in Vitamin A, C, B-complex
-Blueberries, blueberry jam, bilberry, burdock root, carrot, black beans, cod liver oil, huckleberries, endive

Specific Remedies:
- Itchy eyes due to contacts: Vitamin B6
- Tired vision due to overuse and strain: blueberries, fresh or in jam or extract
- Blurred vision: longan fruit

Orthomolecular Considerations
-Lutein
-Omega 3/6 Fatty Oils

Phytotherapeutic Considerations
- Dusty Miller: weak vision due to constitutional or acute conditions
- Eyebright: as a compress relieves redness, swelling and visual disturbance in acute and subacute inflammation, and fresh eye injuries
- Bilberry fruit: especially with diabetic retinopathy, macular degeneration or retinal inflammation.
- Chamomile
- Chrysanthemum
- Rue
- Black Cohosh
- Seneca Snakeroot

Environmental Considerations
- Exposure to fluorescent lights
- Reading in poor (dim) lighting
- Environmental allergens
- Chlorine in swimming pools
- Air conditioning and forced hot air or baseboard heating

Somatic Therapies:
-Vision therapy
-Eye exercises
-Qigong exercises for nourishing the eyes – pressure with thumb and index finger, intensifying when exhaling and decreasing when inhaling. Massage with circular movements both clockwise and counterclockwise: BL-1, BL-2, Yu Yao, TW-23, GB-1, ST-1, ST-2, LI-20, GB-14, Tai Yang, GB-20, LI-4

Acupuncture/Acupresuure/Tapping Considerations

General Local Acupuncture Points with Significance to Eye Diseases			
Point	Effect on Eye Diseases	Point	Effect on Eye Diseases
BL-1	Meeting point of Yin Qiao and Yang Qiao Mai; clears vision, disperses wind, clears heat, opens network vessels	GB-17	Meeting point with Yang Wei Mai, disperses wind
BL-2	Clears vision, disperses wind, opens the network vessels	GB-18	Meeting point with Yang Wei Mai, disperses wind and wind-heat, regulates Liver Qi
BL-3	Disperses wind	GB-20	Meeting point with Yang Wei Mai and Yang Qiao Mai, disperses wind, clears heat, clears vision
BL-6	Disperses wind, transforms	ST-1	Meeting point with Yang Qiao

163

	dampness, eliminates "eye screens"		Mai and Ren Mai, disperses wind, leaches out wind-heat, clears vision
BL-7	Disperses wind, relaxes spasms, dissipates wind-dampness blockages	ST-2	Disperses wind, clears vision, regulates the Liver
BL-8	Strengthens and raises Liver Qi, disperses wind, opens the network vessels	ST-3	Meeting point with Yang Qiao Mai, disperses wind, leaches out wind-heat, supports Liver Qi, moves Blood
BL-10	Disperses wind, opens the network vessels, transforms dampness	ST-4	Meeting point with Yang Qiao Mai and Ren Mai, calms internal wind
SI-18	Disperses wind diseases	ST-8	Meeting point with Yang Wei Mai, disperses wind, supports and regulates Liver and Gallbladder
TW-17	Clears vision, disperses wind	GV-16	Meeting point with Yang Wei Mai, disperses wind, relaxes spasms
TW-20	Eliminates "eye screens" and spasms, leaches out wind-dampness	GV-17	Supports and regulates Liver and Spleen, disperses wind, leaches out damp-heat
TW-22	Supports the Qi, disperses wind, leaches out dampness	GV-19	Disperses wind, regulates Liver Qi
TW-23	Moves the Blood, regulates Qi, disperses wind	GV-20	Meeting point with all Yang and Liver meridians, opens orifices, supports and regulates Liver, disperses wind, directs Liver Yang downward, directs true Yang upward
GB-1	Connection to divergent channels of the Liver, clears vision, disperses wind and wind-heat	GV-21	Disperses wind, leaches out wind-heat
GB-3	Disperses wind, relaxes spasms	GV-23	Leaches out wind-heat
GB-5	Regulates Qi, disperses wind, clears heat	GV-24	Disperses wind, directs flaring Yang downward
GB-7	Apopoletic symptoms	Yintang	Disperses wind and heat, sedates
GB-8	Disperses phlegm blockages, leaches out wind and wind-dampness	Taiyang	Clears the eyes, leaches out wind and wind-heat, clears heat
GB-12	Regulates Liver Qi, leaches out	Yu Yao	Leaches out wind and wind-

164

	wind and wind-heat			heat, clears vision
GB-14	Meeting Point with Yang Wei Mai, clears vision, disperses wind		Qiu Hou	Dissipates internal blockages, clears vision
GB-15	Meeting point with Yang Wei Mai, disperses wind, supports and regulates Liver and Gallbladder		Yi Ming	Clears vision, calms the Shen
GB-16	Meeting point with Yang Wei Mai, disperses wind, regulates Liver and Gallbladder			

Floaters

Floaters occur within the vitreous fluid of the eye behind the retina. They appear as black dots, strands, or squiggles in one's visual field. As the net-like structure of collagen fibers deteriorates over time they may tangle or clump together to create "fibrils". Floaters are the result of shadows on the retina from encountering irregularities in the gelatinous matrix that is the vitreous fluid. They may be especially visible when one is looking at a plain, well-lit background. A sudden vitreous shrinkage, which can happen with age due to drying and thickening, can cause a pulling away from the retina and the appearance of substantial floaters. Floaters tend to occur more frequently in those with myopia or diabetes.

Symptoms:
-Dryness and discomfort of the eyes
-Distending pain
-Dizziness
-Vexation and nausea after extensive work at close distances (reading, computer work, etc.)
-Symptoms may resolve with rest

Biomedical Approach
-None. Virectomies are available for more severe cases

Natural Treatment Approaches
Dietary Considerations
-proteins: emphasize fish, soy, almonds, sunflower seeds, sesame seeds
        avoid: red meat, poultry, dairy
-brown rice with whole grains instead of processed grains such as white bread or pasta
-lots of vegetables
        avoid: nightshade family (tomatoes, green peppers, eggplant)
-steam or bake foods instead of frying
-drink primarily water (8 glasses/day)
-minimize salt

Orthomolecular Considerations

-Omega-3 fatty acids
-Vitamin A
-Vitamin C – strengthens connective tissue of the eye, <1500mg daily to prevent malabsorption of other mineral
-Vitamin E
-Beta-carotene
-Selenium
-Chromium – deficiency increases risk 8 fold
-Glucosamine sulfate - repairs and rebuilds connective tissues to prevent detachment
-Lutein
-Spirulina, chlorella, blue-green algae

Phytotherapeutic Considerations
-Ginkgo biloba
-Chysanthemum (tea or compress)
-Grapeseed extract
-Bilberry

Amblyopia

The conventional definition of amblyopia is reduced vision resulting in disuse of the eye. It is not a turned or wandering eye, but that may be the consequence of either of these problems. If a person's eye becomes misaligned (for example crossed in or turned out) the brain may selectively ignore the image coming from the turned eye. In time, the nervous pathways from the eye to the brain become underdeveloped and a lazy eye develops.

Amblyopia is not an optical problem but a problem involving the pathway from the eye to the visual cortex of the brain. Although amblyopia is commonly called "lazy eye", the eye in this condition is not really lazy. It simply has not received proper stimulation for some of the following reasons

1) The eye has a prescription much different from the other eye. This makes it hard for the visual cortex of the brain to integrate the two images. If this happens before the age of six, visual development will not proceed normally.

2) One eye turns in, out or up at all times and the problem begins before age six. When the two eyes are not able to align on a target, the child will initially experience double vision. As double vision is intolerable to the brain, one of the adaptations to help eliminate it is to reduce vision in the turned eye so that the brain will learn to ignore it.

Amblyopia generally does not develop once the visual system has matured (after age 8 or 9) without some external trauma.

Conventional Treatment
A patch is prescribed for the "good" or normal eye, requiring the "lazy" eye to be used. It is then made stronger out of necessity. The extent and duration of the patching depends on the age of the individual, the severity of the condition, and the response to treatment. Dilating

the pupil of the normal eye is used in occasional cases where patching cannot be done.

Methods to correct the underlying abnormality that may also correct the lazy eye include:
-Eye muscle surgery
-Vision therapy
-Prescription glasses
-Lid surgery.

Natural Treatment Approaches
Dietary Considerations
Vision dietary recommendations

Orthomolecular Considerations
-Lutein

Phytotherapeutic Considerations
-Billberry
-Multi-green formula

Exercises
-Qigong eye exercises

Myopia
In myopia, objects at close distances are seen more clearly than objects at far distances. It is believed to happen secondarily to an excessive curvature of the cornea and/or a longer-than-normal eyeball. In myopia, instead of focusing on the retina in the area called the fovea, the light focuses in front of the retina. This results in the image appearing blurred for objects at a distance.

Myopia affects more than 80 million people in the United States. The majority of people who develop nearsightedness do so within the first 18 years of life. By age 10 about 10% of people are nearsighted; by age 18 it increases to 40% of the population. The degree of near sightedness can vary, as can the age of onset and rate of progression. Nearsightedness does not develop suddenly, but slowly over time. Most nearsighted individuals develop symptoms by the age of eight or nine and progress over the next ten years, stabilizing by the late teens or early twenties.

Genetic predisposition, malnutrition or various syndromes such as Down's Syndrome or ophthalmological diseases can be factors. Environmental factors can play a role as well - the increasing percentages above correspond very well to the increasing close-to face work required in school. As an individual reads more or does more work on a computer or smart phone, the ciliary muscles of the eyes that control the focusing of the eye work harder to focus at these near distances. As they do this for longer and longer periods of time, the muscles find it hard to relax into a position that allows focus at a distance.

Symptoms
-Blurred sight at a distance.
-Generally affects both sides but one may be worse

-Sight tends to be worse at night.
-Early signs of myopia tend to occur in the child who has his or her face in the book for long periods of time without ever looking up. That child might experience some blurring at distance as he or she looks up and finds it takes longer to get far-away objects into focus.

Biomedical Approaches
-Glasses or contacts are prescribed to correct the refraction error – concave lenses
-Laser refractive surgery

Natural Treatment Approaches
Dietary Considerations
Vision dietary recommendations

Orthomolecular Considerations
-Calcium
-Magnesium
-Phosphorus
-Zinc
-Lutein

Phytotherapeutic Considerations
-Billberry
-Multi-green formula

Hyperopia (farsightedness)
This refractive condition is due to either a smaller-than-normal length of the eye or a relatively flat curvature of the cornea. In hyperopia, objects at far distances are seen more clearly than those at in close proximity. The amount of farsightedness can vary with age. It can be overcome somewhat by strengthening the focusing power of the lens to help see near objects clearly.

Hyperopia is normal in newborn and young children and tends to lessen as children get older.

Symptoms
-Blurred vision
-Eyestrain or headaches when looking at near objects

Conventional Treatment
Glasses are prescribed to correct the refractive error

Natural Treatment Approaches
Dietary Considerations
Vision dietary recommendations

Orthomolecular Considerations
-Lutein
-Omega 3 fatty Acids

Phytotherapeutic Considerations
-Bilberry
-Multi-Green Formula

Astigmatism

Conventional theory is that astigmatism is caused by an irregularity in the shape of the cornea (and/or lens) of the eye in which it becomes more oblong, or "football shaped", rather than round. This distorts the light entering the eye and creates a blurred image on the retina. Astigmatism is quite common and frequently occurs along with near-sightedness and farsightedness. It usually affects both sides but can only affect one. Like other visual conditions, astigmatism is not necessarily a fixed entity. Keeping one's head held to the side for long periods of time (such as musicians) has shown changes in astigmatism due to the chronic straining of some eye muscles while relaxing others.

Symptoms
-Blurred, distorted vision at near, distance or both, depending on the amount of astigmatism
-May involve symptoms of eye strain such as headaches, dizziness, blurred vision, eye redness and twitching
-Straight lines may appear crooked, lines may be clearer in one direction than another

Conventional Treatment
-Glasses or contacts are prescribed if vision is impaired or eye strain present
-Refractive surgery

Natural Treatment Approaches

Phytotherapeutic Considerations
Lutein
Billberry
Multi-green formula

Strabismus

Two Types:
- Paralytic (noncomitant)
- Nonparalytic (comitant or concomitant)

Symptoms:
- Acute double vision
- Oculomotor nerve palsy: drooping eyelid, deviation of eye out and down, pupil may be involved
- Trochlear nerve palsy: affected eye deviates up and out
- Abducens nerve palsy: limited abduction of affected eye
- May occur unilaterally or bilaterally
- Compensatory head posturing

Etiology:

- Paralytic: may follow defects in oculomotor nuclei, nerves or muscles; may be caused by CNS, thyroid, muscle diseases, congenital abnormalities, trauma, neoplasm, infection
- Nonparalytic: muscles function but do not properly converge; may follow vision problems, especially pediatric hyperopia
- Some physicians have noted mild strabismus associated with anxiety states in young people, particularly in anorexic/bulimic types.

Biomedical Treatment Approaches
-Ophthalmological treatment depending on clinical findings
        -Conservative
        -Surgical

Natural Treatment Approaches
Somatic Considerations
-eye exercises: can include patching of strong eye

Chapter 23
Sleep Disturbances

Approximately 30-70% of individuals in surveys who have experienced a brain injury have reported sleep disturbances following their injury. These may include post-traumatic excessive sleeping (hypersomnia), narcolepsy, apnea, periodic limb movement disorder and insomnia. Often this dysregulation of the body's daily cycles and lack of proper time to rest and rejuvenate its resources can worsen other symptoms such as pain, irritability and cognitive or mood problems.

Multiple brain centers for sleep and wakefulness have been identified. The brain stem, basal forebrain and hypothalamus regulate the normal sleep-wake cycle. The neurotransmitters serotonin and acetylcholine are involved in this process, as are other internally made products such as dopamine, and norepinephrine. The sleep-wake cycle is also regulated by the interactions of internal synchronizers, or "biological clocks", stemming from the hypothalamus. External factors that synchronize the body include changes in light-darkness, eating and social schedule, temperature and relative humidity. Cognitive deficits and/or sensory deprivation may further impact disorders of sleep in individuals with brain injury.

A study of individuals with moderate to severe TBI showed low cerebrospinal fluid levels of hypocretin 1, a neuropeptide known to be low or absent in those with narcolepsy. These decreased levels were associated with a lower level of arousal. Individuals with TBI were also shown to have an increase in slow wave sleep and reduced REM sleep that resulted in waking frequently at night.

It has been suggested that sleep complaints may vary over time. Difficulty falling and staying asleep tends to occur soon after injury, whereas excessive daytime sleepiness occurs months or years after injury. Post-injury anxiety has been demonstrated to be the most consistent risk factor for worsening sleep.

There are two distinct states of sleep. Rapid Eye Movement, or REM sleep, occurs every 90-100 minutes and lasts anywhere from 10-40 minutes. This state consists of increased brain and physiological activity similar to that of wakefulness. Non-rapid eye movement sleep is a more restful, peaceful state with three stages as outlined in the table below.

Sleep States	
Rapid Eye Movement	Non-rapid eye movement
-High level of brain activity -Physiological activity akin to waking state -Episodic bursts of rapid eye movement -Dreaming with vivid dream recall -Inability to regulate body heat -Absence of body movement -Increase in pulse rate, blood pressure, and respiratory rate	-Low level of brain activity -Physiological activity markedly reduced -No rapid eye movement activity -Three stages present with arousal threshold lowest in stage 1 and highest in stage 3 -Hypothermia -Slight decrease in pulse rate, blood pressure, and respiratory rate

-EEG reveals low voltage mixed-frequency waves	-Decrease in blood flow through all tissues -Intermittent involuntary body movement -EEG reveals increased-voltage, slowed-frequency waves

Stages of non-rapid eye movement sleep	
Stage	General Characteristics
1	Light stage of sleep, lasts briefly Slow eye movement Occupies approximately 5% of sleep Hypnic jerks are common If aroused feel they have been awake
2	Occupies approximately 50% of sleep No eye movement Dreaming very rare Easily awakened
3	Slow wave sleep Disorganization during arousal Dreaming more common than other stages Stages most often involving parasomnias (e.g sleepwalking, somniloquy, night terrors, sleep paralysis)

Post-Traumatic Hypersomnia
This is a disorder in which there is excessive sleeping as a result of a traumatic event involving the central nervous system.

Key characteristics are:
-Excessive sleepiness
-Cognitive or physical fatigue

These may worsen over time as the individual gets farther out from the time of injury. Naps are generally not refreshing or effective in feeling sleepy. No differences have been found between those experiencing hypersomnia and those who do not in various factors including Glasgow Coma Scale score, length of coma, time since brain injury, nature of injury, gender, or medications.

Narcolepsy
While less common, narcolepsy can develop after a brain injury.

This is typically characterized by:
-Catalepsy – sudden loss of muscle tone whereby one will suddenly collapse into sleep
-Hypnagogic hallucinations – vivid dream-like visual, auditory or tactile sensations between waking and sleep states
-Repeated episodes of naps or lapses into sleep for short periods (10-20 minutes)

172

The individual will often begin to feel sleepy again after about 2 to 3 hours, repeating the cycle. Generally the individual's consciousness will remain clear, breathing intact, and their memory will not be affected by cataleptic episodes which can last from a few seconds to several minutes.

Central and Deep Apnea
Obstructive sleep apnea syndrome is characterized by repetitive episodes of upper airway obstruction during sleep. Is is usually associated with reduction in blood oxygen levels. Loud snoring or brief gasps can often accompany this condition with silent periods of approximately 20-30 seconds. Cardiac arrhythmias commonly occur during sleep. Slow heart rate (bradycardia) can also occur during sudden halting of breathing (apnea). Hypertension may also occur.

Central sleep apnea is a decreasing or stopping of breathing during sleep and is associated with lowered oxygen levels in the blood. It appears to be related to changes in the feedback loop between the lungs and the brain. An individual may appear restless as well as gasping, grunting or choking during sleep.

Periodic Limb Movement Disorder
This involves periodic episodes of repetitive limb movements that happen during sleep. Most often this is in the legs, with extension of the first toe and partial flexion of the ankle, knee, and sometimes hip. While less common, similar movements can happen in the upper limbs. They can even occur when an individual is partially awake or waking up. Someone may not even be aware of these movements and simply describe waking frequently throughout the night, or of restless sleep.

Approaches to this condition can include proper hydration (as dehydration can be a factor), magnesium supplementation (internal or topical), or *Bai Shao Gan Cao Wan* – a simple formula consisting of white peony root and licorice root.

Insomnia
Insomnia is the most common sleep disturbance reported by those affected by brain injury. Literature suggests that more than 80% of those with a TBI complain of poor sleep and daytime sleepiness.

Key components of insomnia include:
-Difficulty falling asleep
-Frequent awakenings with difficulty falling back asleep (over 30 minutes)
-Feeling of fatigue throughout the day

In order to meet the requirements for insomnia established in the DSM-V, the sleep disturbance must last for more than a month and happen more than twice per week. It is suggested that most cases do not tend to subside over time following the injury. It has been shown that those who were found to have high anxiety scores had more trouble falling asleep, while those with high depression scores had more difficulty maintaining sleep. Pain is also closely associated with insomnia.

Diagnosis
-Self-reporting

-Polysomnography (PSG)
-Mutliple Sleep Latency Test (MSLT)
-Actigraphy

Biomedical Approaches
Benzodiazepine Hypnotics
        -Lorazepam
        -Temazepam
        -Clonazepam (Klonopin)
        -Triazolam
Nonbenzodiazepine Sedative-hypnotics
        -Zolpidem (Ambien)
        -Zaleplon (Sonata)
        -Eszopiclone (Prosom)
Antidepressants
        -Trazedone
        -Amitriptyline
Antipsychotics
        -Risperidone (insomnia and psychosis)
        -Quetiapine (insomnia with paranoia or agitation)
-C-PAP or bi-level pressure oral appliances (sleep apnea)
-Modafinil (sleep apnea, narcolepsy)
-Melatonin
-Phototherapy
-Chronotherapy

Natural Treatment Approaches

Dietary Considerations:
therapeutic foods:
- Increase foods that calm the Shen (Spirit), tonify the Heart, harmonize the Stomach and Spleen
- Foods high in tryptophan: nuts, eggs, meat, fish, dairy
- If supplementing tryptophan: give with cofactors (Vitamins B3, B6, and C) and whole wheat toast, bananas, walnuts, pineapples that are high in serotonin
-Increase foods high in Vitamin C, Vitamin B-complex

avoid: meat, alcohol, hot sauces, spicy foods, fried foods, fatty foods, rich foods, salty foods, coffee, caffeine, sweet foods and sugar

Somatic Therapies:
- Aerobic exercise program (20 minutes per day)
- Nourish breathing: before bed
- Qigong
- Tai qi chuan
- Progressive relaxation/guided meditation

Just before bedtime, do the following exercise of contracting then relaxing your muscles:

While lying down, take 5 or 6 deep, slow breaths. Then tighten up the muscles of your face and neck into an ugly grimace for about 2 seconds. Then let go and relax. Then hunch your shoulders and tighten up the muscles of your arms. Let go and relax. Follow this pattern with the stomach muscles, legs, and then feet and toes. Then contract all the muscles of your body and relax. Repeat this whole sequence 2 or 3 more times, putting attention on deep breathing.

Phytotherapeutic Considerations
The following herbs used alone or in combination can help to induce quality sleep without producing the groggy, hard-to-awaken feeling the next morning that is common with sleeping pills:
-Red date seed (Suan Zao Ren)
-Chamomile
- Hops
- Passion Flower
- Skullcap
- Valerian (which is a strong sedative)

If used as a tea, combine 1 tablespoon of herb per cup of boiling water. Steep 20 minutes and drink 1/2 hour before bedtime. If used as a tincture (liquid herbal extract), 30 to 60 drops of any combination are taken with a little water.

Orthomolecular Considerations
-Tryptophan (3-5g)
-5-HTP (100-300mg)
-Melatonin (3mg)
-Niacin (100mg, decrease if "flushing" occurs)
-Vitamin B6 (50mg)
-Magnesium (250mg)
-Phosphorus
-Lithium (Anxiousness)

Clinical Notes:
-While the use of melatonin as a natural sleep aid can be beneficial, it is important to note that it is a hormone secreted by the pineal gland in response to fluctuations in light and darkness. Long term and consistent supplementation of melatonin can establish an artificial external source of the hormone, making the body less likely to consistently produce it on its own. Strong consideration should be given to utilizing melatonin either in the short term or in short periods followed by a brief break from supplementation. This may be taking it 2-3 days then taking a day off or supplementing for a week then taking 2-3 days off to allow the body to continue natural production.

Acupressure/Tapping Considerations
PC-6, Yintang, HT-8, BL-47, An Mian, Ear Shenmen

Nightmares/Night Terrors

Differential Diagnosis:
Medical Disorders:
      -Narcolepsy
      -Epilepsy
      -Seizure Disorders
Psychiatric Disorders:
      -Anxiety disorders
      -Schizophrenia and other psychotic disorders
      -Post-Traumatic Stress Disorder (PTSD)

Natural Treatment Approaches

Dietary Considerations:
therapeutic foods:
-Increase foods that calm the Shen, tonify the Heart, harmonize the Stomach and Spleen

avoid:
-Meat, alcohol, hot sauces, spicy foods, fried foods, fatty foods, rich foods, salty foods, coffee, caffeine, sweet foods and sugar, processed foods
- Refined carbohydrate, food allergens

Phytotherapeutic Considerations
Red Date Seed (Suan Zao Ren)
Lavender
Passionflower
Skullcap
Peony seed (powdered)
Pasque flower
Swamp Verbena
Hops (use as small stuffed pillow)
Mugwort (under pillow – folk remedy)

Acupressure/Tapping Considerations
Ear Shenmen, GB-40, BL-47

Somnolence/Hypersomnia

Etiology
- Lowering of basal metabolic rate accompanying hypothyroidism
- Central nervous system injuries affecting the hypothalamus or brain stem which disrupt normal functioning of the brain circuits that permit normal sleep.
- Chronic abuse of marijuana, heroin, opioids, and other CNS depressants
-Psychopharmacological agents including many antidepressants and some OTC medications have significant sedating effects
-Dysregulation of serotonin, norepinephrine, or other neurotransmitters in depression

Differential Diagnosis
Medical Disorders
      -Hypothyroidism
      -Hypothalamic Lesions
      -Seizure Disorders
      -Diffuse Axonal Injury
Effects of Substances
      -Alcohol or illicit substance intoxication or withdrawal
      -Side effects of medications
Psychiatric Disorders
      -Depressions
      -Bipolar Disorder, Depressive Phase

Natural Treatment Approaches
See chapter 10 on approaches to fatigue

Chapter 24
Impaired Attention/Concentration

Impairment in attention is a very common occurrence following a brain injury regardless of level of severity. Common symptoms include mental slowing, trouble following conversation, loss of train of thought, and difficulty in attending to more than one thing at once. The degree of change following a brain injury reflect multiple factors including severity of diffuse axonal injury, length of amnesia, extent of atrophy, and the location and depth of the injury. Age, pre-existing conditions, genetic factors and any additional bodily injuries such as low oxygen or low blood pressure can also be factors.

The early phases of recovery and post-traumatic amnesia can show signs of impaired awareness and wandering attention. Even mild injury can restrict processes such as the ability to learn new information due to the ability to maintain attention playing into all aspects of cognition.

The concept of attention can be subdivided into categories of selective, sustained, and divided attentions. Information processing speed and supervisory (or executive) aspects of attention are also considered.

The brainstem reticular formation supports overall tone of attention and degree of responsiveness. The right hemisphere is believed to have a greater role in sustained attention, while the left hemisphere may be more closely linked to selective and focused attention. Selective attention has also been attributed to the functioning of the posterior parietal, dorsolateral frontal, and cingulate regions of the brain, working in conjunction with the thalamus, basal ganglia, and midbrain.

Often a slowed reaction time is proportionate to complexity of the task being performed. This is particularly true when needing to decide between several choices. Slowed processing time has been theorized to be responsible for many concerns of attention. Limitations in executive control over attention has been thought to govern lower-level attentional processes including allocation of attention resources, target selection, interference control, shifting between tasks, monitoring, etc.

Attention Subtypes	
Focused	Perceive and respond to internal and external events. Selection of one source of information while not attending to irrelevant information
Sustained	Maintain attention to complete a task accurately and efficiently over a period of time
Selective	Maintain attention in the presence of distractions
Alternating	Shift focus between tasks demanding different behavioral or cognitive skills
Divided	Respond simultaneously in multiple task demands while maintaining speed and accuracy

179

Other domains of cognitive functioning that may be affected by brain injury
Categorization: Ability to identify objects based on attributes (e.g. color, shape, construction, size, texture, detail, function)
Memory: Consolidation, storage and recall of information
Processing Speed: Speed at which information is processed
Executive Functions: Planning, reasoning, judgment, initiation and abstract thinking, problem solving, decision making
Metacognition: Self awarenes and knowledge of one's strengths and weaknesses

Biomedical Approaches
Cholinergic Agents
    -Physostigmine
    -Cytidine-5-diphosphocholine
    -Cholinesterase inhibitors (donepezil, rivastigmine, galantamine)
Catecholaminergic Agents
    -Psychostimulants (methylphenidate, dextroamphetamine)
    -Amantadine
    -Bromocriptine
    -Levodopa
    -Selegiline
Other Agents
    -Tricyclic antidepressants
    -Other antidepressants – SSRI's, SNRI's, bupropion
    -Atomoxetine (SNRI)
    -Dopamine receptor agonists: Pergolide, pramipexole, ropinirole
    -Guanfacine
    -Lamotrigine
    -Memantine
Attention Processing Training (APT) – Tasks are organized by increasing difficulty, and progression to a higher skill level occurs when the easier task is mastered. Repetition of a task results in a reduction in the amount of effort and attention control required

Natural Treatment Approaches
Lifestyle Considerations
-If easily distracted: never do more than one thing at a time
-If unable to multi-task: Repeatedly check and work to regain attention
-If very short attention span: Work in a quiet and closed environment. For some music may be helpful in maintaining attention while for others it may be a distractor.

Dietary Considerations
Diet can at times have a significant impact on attentional concerns, particularly if a food allergy or sensitivity is present.
therapeutic foods:
- Whole-foods diet, high in protein and complex carbohydrates; reduce sugar and simple carbohydrates.
- Increase foods that calm the Shen (Spirit), tonify the Heart, harmonize the Stomach and Spleen

- Increase foods rich in Vitamin B-complex
- Longan, oyster, rice, rosemary, wheat, wheat germ, mushroom (maitake, shiitake, reishi)

Avoid:
- Food additive sensitivities: eliminate processed foods that contain artificial colors, flavors, sweeteners, and preservatives, commonly listed as benzoates, nitrates, and sulfites; common food additives also include calcium silicate, BHT, BHA, benzoyl peroxide, emulsifiers, thickeners, stabilizers, vegetable gums, and food starch.

-Minimize food sensitivities: eliminate or reduce the intake of cow's milk, soy, eggs, wheat, citrus, and other potential allergenic foods

- Minimize sugars and simple carbohydrates to reduce risk of hypoglycemic reactions:
-avoid meat, alcohol, hot sauces, spicy foods, fried foods, fatty foods, rich foods, salty foods, coffee, caffeine, sweet foods and sugar

Chinese Nutritional Approach:
-Heart Blood Deficiency, Spleen Qi Deficiency, and Yin Deficiency, Yang hyperactivity: nourishing, cooked, warm, clear bland diet, with slightly increased animal protein to help manufacture sufficient blood, for example, soups with black beans, chicken or beef broth, and plentiful root and leafy green vegetables

- Phlegm Obstructing the Heart Orifices: avoid Sweet, Cold and Damp foods which either weaken the Spleen, such as chilled, cold, raw foods or sugar and sweets, or foods which cause Dampness and Phlegm, such as sugar and sweets, dairy foods, and fatty, greasy, fried foods

- Heat Excess: eliminate all food additives, colorings and flavorings; avoid oranges, sugar and red meat, as well as hot foods such as hot spices, shellfish and curries

- Heat and Phlegm: eliminate Phlegm-producing foods such as dairy and peanut butter; high frequency of gluten intolerance which causes green phlegm and nasal congestion; avoid Sweet and Damp foods

- Middle Jiao Deficiency, including Spleen Qi Deficiency: limit sweets and fruit juices, especially restrict cold food and drinks; no ice

- Kidney Qi Deficiency: limit sweets and cold food; no ice

Somatic Therapy Considerations
- Gentle exercise
- Eurhythmy
- Yoga
- Qigong

Orthomolecular Considerations
-B-Complex
-Iron
-Zinc
-Magnesium

181

-Essential fatty acids

Phytotherapeutic Considerations
-Polygonum (Yuan Zhi)
-Black Cohosh
-Chamomile
-Wild Oat
-California Poppy
-Evening Primrose
-Siberian Ginseng
-Hops
-Oatstraw
-St. John's Wort
-Lavender
-Melissa
-Passionflower
-Skullcap
-Valerian

Acupressure/Tapping Considerations
-GV-16, GV-20, PC-5, PC-7, Si Shen Cong

Chapter 25
Memory Impairment and Dementia

Memory dysfunction is considered a flagship feature following a brain injury. During the acute recovery phase, retrograde amnesia and post-traumatic amnesia can certainly have a strong impact. Memory complaints in the post-acute phase can often persist as well. In cases of mild TBI most symptoms tend to resolve within 1-3 weeks following the injury. In moderate to severe injuries symptoms may persist. A brain injury can effect any part of memory functioning – encoding, storage, or retrieval of information may all be impacted. The transferring of information from short-term to long-term memory, a process known as consolidation, can also influenced. In order for information to become encoded it must be present and attended to, allowing for storage. The information must be stored in order to be later retrieved. As such, a dysfunction anywhere in this process will cause memory impairments.

Those who have experienced a brain injury may test worse in memory tasks such as recalling a list of 15 words presented to them (either visually or auditory) than those with no such injury.

The different types of memory are as follows:
Sensory Memory: Holds a memory of sensory input for a matter of a few seconds. This allows the screening of large amounts of information and can be vulnerable to "washout". The five forms of sensory memory relate to the five senses: auditory, visual, smell, touch, and taste.

Short-Term Memory: Information recall lasts for a few minutes to hours. Information is passively held. Some psychologists consider short-term memory and working memory interchangeable terms, others consider them separate functions.

Working Memory: Active, rather than passive, this is a temporary storage of information in order to accomplish a task.

Long-Term Memory: Permanent consolidation and storage of information that may remain a lifetime. Long-term memory can be further divided into either explicit, which can be consciously recalled, or implicit memory, which is a unconscious procedural process.

Examples of explicit memory – general knowledge/facts about the world (semantic memory), personal recollection of experiences (episodic memory)

Examples of implicit memory – procedural memory (e.g. "muscle memory", tying shoes, riding a bike), cognitive skill memory (e.g. procedures needed to solve a problem or win a game), classical conditioning

Aspects of memory relating to executive function
-Working memory
-Strategic memory: active organizing strategies to enhance encoding and retrieval
-Source memory: context for episodic memory: where, when, and time order

-Prospective memory: remembering to perform a task in the future at a certain time
-Metamemory: awareness and knowledge of one's memory abilities

Episodic memory impairment is a hallmark feature of a TBI and generally corresponds to the severity of the injury.

Working memory can also often be affected where processing and manipulating information has been linked to the dorsolateral prefrontal lobe. This also corresponds to updating stored information, inhibiting unwanted thoughts, and the ability to shift between verbal and visual information. Organizing strategies during learning such as word categorization (e.g. "vegetables", "cars") has often been shown to be affected.

If prospective memory is affected, someone may fail to effectively gauge the severity of their memory impairment, believing they perform better than they actually do. This shows a deficit in self-awareness of one's abilities (metamemory).

A traumatic brain injury tends to effect the brain's control/manipulation processes more than the passive storage/rehearsal aspects. Recognition memory tends to remain intact, as does implicit memory.

MRI findings have consistently shown atrophy in the hippocampus following injury. This, coupled with the hippocampus being particularly sensitive to injury, strongly implicates the hippocampus (and entorhinal cortex) as crucial structures in problems of explicit memory. The hippocampus is assumed to protect memory and the encoding of new information during the storage and consolidation phase by filtering/exclusion/dampening irrelevant and interfering information. When the hippocampus is damaged, input overload can result as the brain becomes overwhelmed by neural noise. This disrupts the consolidation phase to where relevant information is not properly stored or even attended to.

Diencephalic and basal forebrain structures are also believed to be strong potential candidates given their substantial role in episodic memory. Mnemonic functioning can be affected by injury to the frontal lobes. Frontal and memory specific temporal networks have also shown to impact attention and executive function memory impairments.

Inferior temporal neurons are involved in both encoding, storage, and recall; and interact with the amygdala and hippocampus in learning, memory and recognition. These inferior neurons are involved in short term emotional, as well as non-emotional, visual and cognitive processing and memory storage. As seen with an injury to the inferior temporal lobe, visual and verbal memory functions may suffer. Electrical stimulation of the inferior and medial temporal lobe have been shown to produce exceedingly vivid personal memories which include such things as complex scenes from early childhood, hearing conversations, seeing faces or experiencing bodily sensations, and related events. Diffuse axonal injury has also been suggested to affect the wider memory networks.

Damage to the left inferior temporal lobe can moderately disrupt immediate memory, and severely impair delayed memory of verbal passages, associations, word lists and number sequences. Right temporal injuries, on the other hand, significantly impair recognition memory for tactile and visual elements such as faces, meaningless designs, and object positioning/orientation. The the front portion of the temporal lobe is more involved in the initial consolidation storage phase of memory while the rear temporal region is involved more with memory retrieval and recall.

The temporal lobes directly interact with the frontal lobes in the process of memorization and remembering. The more active these areas are, the more likely someone will remember, whereas reduced activity is associated with forgetting. Thus, if the frontal lobe is injured, even if the temporal lobes are not, someone may have significant memory loss due to an inability to correctly search for and find the memory.

Biomedical Treatments
Cholinergic Agents
       -Physostigmine
       -Cytidine-5-diphosphocholine
       -Cholinesterase inhibitors (donepezil, rivastigmine, galantamine)
Catecholaminergic Agents
       -Psychostimulants (methylphenidate, dextroamphetamine)
       -Amantadine
       -Bromocriptine
       -Levodopa
       -Selegiline
Other Agents
       -Tricyclic antidepressants
       -Other antidepressants – SSRI's, SNRI's, bupropion)
       -Atomoxetine (SNRI)
       -Dopamine receptor agonists: Pergolide, pramipexole, ropinirole
       -Guanfacine
       -Lamotrigine
       -Memantine
-Improving attention, perception and categorization skills
-External compensatory strategies – alarms, memory notebooks, digital devices

Dementia

Dementia may be caused by structural damage to brain tissue or can result as a progressive decline in intellectual function that interferes substantially with the person's normal social or economic activities. A single brain trauma with diffuse injury to the tissue may incite dementia. Dementia can also develop as the result of multiple mild TBIs in which Chronic Traumatic Encephalopathy (CTE) occurs. CTE is a rare, progressive, and degenerative condition of the central nervous system which typically follows repetitive brain trauma. This may be due to high risk sports such as football or boxing. In this case, diffuse axonal injury causes a release of Tau proteins which are changed structurally by metabolic breakdown of brain cells to create a chronic inflammatory state that causes a progressive degeneration of the central nervous system.

Etiology and classification

May occur at any age, from any injury, in which enough impact is sustained to cause widespread damage to associative brain areas

185

Static dementia
-Stems from single major injury (severe head injury) - nonprogressive

Progressive dementias
-Alzheimer's Disease: brain atrophy, degenerative loss of cells, acetylcholine neurons affected, senile plaques, neurofibrillary tangles, abnormally increased proteins in brain.
Major components: Heart disease of any kind, hypertension, diabetes, obesity.
Some are now calling this a "type 3 diabetes" due to evidence of blood sugar correlates.

-Unknown cause (idiopathic), or simple, presenile dementia: Alzheimer-like changes, multiple injuries, age of onset is abnormal

-Multi-infarct dementia: small and large injuries to the brain due to stroke, clotting, or bleeding of varying age, step-wise intellectual dysfunction, neurological symptoms, depression

-AIDS dementia: late stage HIV with cognitive, emotional, motor deficits

-Chronic traumatic encephalopathy (CTE): progressive dementia from repeated head injury

Degrees of Severity
-Mild Cognitive Impairment: memory problems better than expected for one's age

-Medium level Alzheimers: Hard to learn new things, difficulty performing tasks that involve multiple steps, impulsivity, paranoid thinking, forgets friends

-Severe Alzheimers: difficulty communicating, does not recognize family, sleeps a lot, loss of bowel/bladder control, lose weight

---

Warning Signs of Dementia

-Asking the same question repeatedly
-Repeating the same story over again - word for word
-Forgetting how to do an activity that used to be easy
-Loss of ability to balance checkbook
-Getting lost and misplacing things
-Neglecting to bathe and wearing the same clothes over and over again
-Reliance on someone else to answer questions and make decisions

---

Signs & Symptoms

-Slow disintegration of personality and intellect	-Difficulty with new skills	-Memory impairment
-Impaired judgment	-Decreased initiative	-Blunted affect
-Loss of affect	-Distractability	-Deteriorated habits
-Depression, paranoia	-Aphasia (speech	-Personality traits exaggerated
-Anxiety	disturbance), apraxia (motor),	-Insidious, progressive
-Restricted interests, difficult	agnosia (recognition of	-Initially more of a problem
conceptual thinking	perceptions)	for family
	-Spatial disorientation	

Diagnosis
- Memory impairment
- Aphasia, apraxia, agnosia, or disturbed executive function
- Continuing cognitive decline

Diagnostic Testing
-Complete Blood Count (CBC)
-Chem screen
-Thyroid function
-Serum B12
-Drug levels
-HIV
-CT Scan
-EEG (wave slowing) -Suggests that the hippocampus is working at a lower level

Differential Diagnosis
- Chronic alcohol use
- Vitamin B12 deficiency
- Drug side-effects
- Primary psychiatric disorder
- Sometimes secondary to a treatable condition

Natural Treatment Approaches

Lifestyle Considerations
-Follow a fixed daily routine
-Write everything down in a working diary
-Repeat every relevant detail throughout the day
-The effects of stress can be reduced through stress management and relaxation techniques such as visualization and meditation. Counseling is strongly encouraged.
- Get adequate rest and take naps as needed.
- Regular physical exercise – at least 30 minutes, 3 times a week. Consultation with a physician about a proper exercise program should be considered if one hasn't exercised for awhile.

Beneficial Activities to Boost Intelligence
-Learn a new language
-Puzzles, crosswords, brain games
-Play a musical instrument
-Listmaking
-New activities and new social environments

Dietary Considerations
-Maintain a healthy diet. This includes using fresh, unprocessed foods. Eat daily servings of leafy green vegetables, whole grains, fresh fruits, and proteins with a minimum of animal fat. Keep intake of sugar foods and refined carbohydrates (such as white bread and white rice) to a minimum.

-Eliminate alcohol, smoking, and drug use.
-Fruit/vegetable juice intake 4-5x/week lowered dementia risk 4x

Phytotherapeutic Considerations
-Ginkgo Biloba - 80 mg TID
-Polygonum (Yuan Zhi)
-Ginseng Root (Ren Shen)
-Huperzine A
-Gotu Kola
-Curcumin/Turmeric
-Green Tea
-Bacopa
-Kempo
-Balm₁
-Sage₁
-Rosemary₁
-Adaptogens: Ashwaghanda, Ginseng, Rhodiola₂

Orthomolecular Considerations
- B-complex vitamin – 50 mg. 3 times per day. Vitamin B deficiency affects brain function.
- Vitamin B12 – 1 milligram per day.
-Vitamin C - 500-1000mg
-Vitamin E - 2,000 IU/day
-Methylcobalamin
- Lecithin – 2 tablespoons per day.
- Glutamic acid – 200 milligrams per day
-Acetyl-L-carnitine - 500 mg TID
-Phosphatidylserine
-Vinpocetine (short term memory)
-Resveratrol
-Pregneneolone
- Niacin – Start with 100 mg. after each meal and increase up to 250 mg. until you feel a flushing of the skin. This stimulates blood circulation to the skin and head. Continue for trial period of 3 weeks. Niacin should only be used only under a doctor's supervision as it can become toxic to the liver after several weeks.

Acupressure/Tapping Considerations
GV-16, GV-20, GV-24, Si Shen Cong

Acupuncture Research Studies
[Di Huang Yin Zi] not only significantly decreased the number of TUNEL-positive cells but also reduced the LDH release of hippocampus of model rats. Morris water maze test showed that the ability of learning and memory of rats dramatically impaired after ischemic brain injury. However, [Di Huang Yin Zi] ameliorated the impairment of learning and memory of ischemic rats. Furthermore, western blotting and immunohistochemical data showed that the expression of extracellular regulated protein and synaptophysin, which correlates with synaptic formation and function, decreased after ischemic insult.

The therapeutic effects of acupuncture plus modified Bu Yang Huan Wu Tang were compared to a pharmaceutical medication in post-stroke cognitive dysfunction. The drug group received 3 tablets of piracetam, three times per day for 8 weeks.. The Chinese medicine group received acupuncture at GB-20 and the extra point Gongxue located 1.5 cun below GB-20 6 days a week and the herbal formula twice daily. The acupuncture plus herbs group achieved a 90% total treatment effective rate. The drug group achieved a 70% total effective rate. Bu Yang Huang Wu Tang was administered in the following modified version: Huang Qi, Dang Gui Wei, Chuan Xiong, Chi Shao, Tao Ren, Hong Hua, Di Long, E Zhu, Shi Chang Pu, Shui Zhi.₁

Chapter 26
Executive Function and Cognition

Executive function collectively refers to some of the most complex cognitive processes the human brain performs. They include:

- Self-awareness
- Planning/Organizing
- Goal setting
- Self-initiation

- Self-monitoring
- Self-evaluation
- Self-inhibition
- Change set

- Strategic behavior
- Working memory

In cases of a brain injury, problems can manifest in the following areas:

- Abstract thought
- Analysis of all aspects of a situation
- Considering all possible solutions to a problem

- Executing solutions
- Mental flexibility if one solution does not work
- Self-monitoring
- Impulsivity

- Disinhibition
- Hyperverbosity
- Lack of emotional control

Executive function deficits can happen at any level of severity and may impact all aspects of daily life. One's interpersonal, social, recreational, emotional, educational, and work life can all be significantly affected. Deficits in executive function are considered a critical determinant of outcomes after a brain injury. Links have been shown between the prefrontal cortex and virtually all other cortical and subcortical regions. Four distinct categories of function have been tied to specific regions of the prefrontal cortex.

Categories of frontal executive function		
Dorsolateral prefrontal cortex	Executive cognitive functions	Spatial, temporal, and conceptual reasoning
Superior medial prefrontal cortex	Activation-regulating functions	Initiating and maintaining mental processes Monitoring response conflict
Ventromedial prefrontal cortex	Behavioral self-regulation functions	Emotional processing Mediation of stimulus-reward associations
Frontal polar regions	Metacognitive processes	Higher-order integrative aspects of personality, self-awareness, and social cognition Prospective memory: complex multitasking

Dorsolateral Prefrontal Cortex:

Injury can result in:
- Difficulties in attention, working memory, planning, and reasoning
- Phonemic and semantic fluency may decline

Diffuse axonal injury may cause executive cognitive functioning deficits whether or not there is direct frontal lobe injury. Higher-order functioning may become apparent or increasingly so in situations where demand or complexity increase.

Tests: verbal fluency tasks (retrieval, monitoring, inhibition), Trail Making Test (part B) (divided attention), Wisconsin Card Sorting Test (concept formation/flexibility)

Superior Medial Prefrontal Cortex: This area plays an important role in initiating and sustaining mental processes at a high enough level to meet goal-directed tasks.

Injury can result in:
-Apathy or abulia (lack of will)
-Milder injuries: slowed reaction time or response on task tests
-Severe cases: mutism and lack of movement.

The superior medial prefrontal cortex is engaged anytime a cognitive task becomes more difficult and demands more monitoring. The anterior cingulate seems to be in play here in monitoring potential conflicts such as in when placed in new, unknown situations. The absence of this activation can contribute to an apathetic state.

Tests: verbal fluency tasks, conflict trial of the Stroop color-naming test

Ventromedial prefrontal cortex: This makes up the limbic portion of the prefrontal cortex and tends to bear the brunt of a traumatic brain injury as it is vulnerable to both focal and diffuse injury.

Injury can result in:
-Lack of insight, impaired planning and decision making
-Social impropriety
-Lack of empathy and dampened or poorly modulated emotional response
-"Social cognition": inability to effectively interpret the behavior of others, make inferences about their feelings, beliefs and intentions, conceptualize one's relationship to another and guide one's behavior based on this information
-Misperception of facial expressions, voice, bodily gestures, social context, and negative emotions such as anger, sadness, disgust and fear (yet not positive emotions) may be deficient.

The ventromedial prefrontal cortex may play a role in such "self-conscious emotions" as embarrassment, shame and pride. There may also be dissociation between unaffected intellectual ability on tests but failure to be able to apply the knowledge in less structured situations. Someone may lack a "gut feeling" due to an inability to process emotionally-related material.

Tests: Iowa Gambling Task (decision-making), Frontal Systems Behavioral Scale

Frontal Poles: This lies in a position to fulfill a specialized, integrative role in relation to the other areas of the prefrontal cortex due to reciprocal connections almost exclusively with higher-order association areas. It receives processed, abstract information from other areas and seems to bridge prefrontal cortex functions with those of emotion, drive and self-regulation.

192

Injury can result in:
-Difficulty with future plans and goals, abstract reward concepts and complex, real world multitasking (having a large overarching goal in mind while achieving smaller independent tasks)
-Difficulty with metacognition (explored below)

Treatment Options
- Cognitive rehabilitation – formal problem solving training with applications in everyday situations and functional routines
- Speech-language pathologists
- Occupational therapists
- Neuropsychologists

Metacognition
This term refers to one's ability to reflect on, and be aware of, their own cognitive functioning. This includes perceived mental acuity that may differ from testing and observation. In other words, one may think they are able to cogitate better than they actually do. Intact metacognition allows someone to be aware of struggles they may experience with problem solving but still not be able to solve the problem. The term for a diminished self-awareness and an inability to recognize personal disability is Anosognosia. Because of this being a higher order cognitive function that reflects upon itself, metacognition has an integrative role for other aspects of executive functioning such as self-monitoring and information processing.

There are three levels of metacognitive impairments:
-Awareness of deficits caused by injury (memory deficits, delays in processing speed, etc.)
-Awareness of functional implications of these deficits
-Awareness to set realistic goals

Treatment Options
Begins with external cues of general rule or principle for solving problems and gradually progress toward an internal, automatic process

 Biomedical Approaches
Cholinergic Agents
        -Physostigmine
        -Cytidine-5-diphosphocholine
        -Cholinesterase inhibitors (donepezil, rivastigmine, galantamine)
Catecholaminergic Agents
        -Psychostimulants (methylphenidate, dextroamphetamine)
        -Amantadine
        -Bromocriptine
        -Levodopa
        -Selegiline
Other Agents
        -Tricyclic antidepressants
        -Other antidepressants – SSRI's, SNRI;s, bupropion)
        -Atomoxetine (SNRI)

-Dopamine receptor agonists: Pergolide, pramipexole, ropinirole
-Guanfacine
-Lamotrigine
-Memantine

Natural Treatment Approaches

Some aspects of cognition have been covered in the previous chapters on memory and attention impairment.

Lifestyle considerations

Bewilderment
-Easily confused or memory gaps and trouble sticking to a schedule: Use a notebook to record and list events and refer to book throughout the day
-Difficulty distinguishing timelines of events: Develop a consistent routine for all tasks. Do not randomly change routines

Indecisiveness
-Write options and pros and cons down in a diary
-Discuss the options in simple terms

Initiation
Either an inability to get into a planned action or lack of interest in activities
-Write down activity and keep a strict daily routine
-Baby steps can make it much easier to get started with the first small step
-Create achievable deadlines

Persistence & perseverance
Tasks are nearly never completed, inability to stick to a plan of action, or a cluttered/ disorganized environment
-Write down the plan and steps to completion in a daily diary
-Develop an interactive checklist
-Start small

Chapter 27
Language and Communication Dysfunction

A study of brain injured individuals 7 years out from a severe injury showed that nearly 50% reported some level of difficulty in speaking. Reports of difficulty in word finding can often follow an injury of any severity level. Communication deficits do tend to accompany moderate to severe injuries however.

Impairments include difficulty in word retrieval, verbal associative fluency, and comprehension of complex auditory input. Conversational aspects can also be affected in which pragmatic use of language like initiating and maintaining a specific topic, attending to the needs of the listener, or using indirect communication such as humor or sarcasm.

Anomic aphasia tends to be the most common form where identifying objects and proper names, and talking in circles (circumlocation) are found. Comprehension and repetition are kept intact. Wernicke's (receptive) aphasia has also been observed, in which the ability to understand language is present. Other forms of aphasias are more rare. Refer to chapter 2 for a more extensive exploration of aphasia.

Other speech disorders such as mutism, stuttering and repetition of speech (echolalia) have also been known to occur. Speech apraxia can be present in which the person cannot effectively translate what they want to say into the ability to initiate speech. Dysarthria, in which muscle weakness impacts the ability to speak, is relatively common following a TBI and can continue to be present after other language problems improve. Many language concerns are considered to have a reasonably good recovery within the first year post-injury, particularly in cases of mild brain injury.

Language and communication dysfunctions cannot be viewed in isolation due to its neural networks linking prefrontal, perisyulvan, and parietal language areas, as well as other regions mediating broader aspects of communication. They reflect the interplay of primary language functions and other non-linguistic processes such as attention, working memory, and higher order executive functions of the prefrontal cortex. Injury of the left prefrontal cortex has been associated with simplified, repetitive and impoverished speech. Right hemisphere prefrontal injury, on the other hand, may show an increase in detail, insertion of irrelevant elements, and a tendency toward socially inappropriate speech.

Differential Diagnosis:
Medical Disorders:
- -Delirium
- -Dementia
- -Cerebrovascular Accident (CVA)
- -Tic Disorders
- -Traumatic Brain Injury
- -Seizure Disorders
- -CNS Tumors

Psychiatric Disorders:

-Schizophrenia and other psychotic disorders
-Acute Mania in Bipolar Disorders or Schizo-affective Disorder
-Pervasive Development Disorders

Natural Treatment Approaches
-Speech-Language Pathologist
-Singing and vocal exercises
-If speaking is difficult, singing the words/phrases may still be possible due to different areas of the brain being used

Lifestyle considerations
Starting a conversation
Lack of response to a conversation, no answering questions, prolonged and inappropriate pauses
-Prompting and attempts to pull someone into a conversation
-Patience and be sure to give someone enough time
-Do not become inattentive

Participating in conversation
Does not understand what is being said, cannot concentrate long enough to follow a discussion, never stops talking, cannot fathom changes in the topic of conversation, difficulty keeping on topic, slurred speech, rapid speech, inaudible or excessively loud speech
-Be concise
-Repeat what is being said if necessary
-Attempt to keep eye contact
-Keep pulling someone back to the conversation by getting their attention
-Interrupt and ask for an opportunity to respond or participate if necessary
-Clarify when new topics are taken on
-Ask the person to repeat until you can make out what they are saying
-Indicate if volume is inappropriate using cues and signals

Body Language
Oblivious to body language cues, disparities between body language and conversation, disconnect between expression and content of communication
-Body language or emotional expression flashcards
-Invades people's personal space: request personal space
- Inappropriate physical contact: express and explain if inappropriate contact happens
-Disruptive movements while talking: ask if they are able to stop any disruptive movements being made
-Ask if expressions do not match their tone or conversational content (e.g. laughing while sad)
-Lack of eye contact or inappropriate looking at or staring at others: Indicate that staring or gaze is inappropriate or ask to make eye contact if appropriate

Acupuncture Research Studies:
-Acupuncture was found effective for the treatment of aphasia after a stroke as patients were found to regain the ability to communicate through speech and written language at a similar rate as drug therapy patients. A combination of acupuncture with drug therapy produced

optimal positive patient outcomes. Acupuncture, as a standalone therapy, produced a 46% total effective rate and donepezfil (a cognition enhancing drug) produced a 50% total effective rate. Significantly, the combination of acupuncture with donepezfil produced a 77% total effective rate. **Points used:** CV-23, GV-15, GV-20, GV-24, Extra Point Laoguan, HT-5, KI-1.[2]

-A 2003 fMRI study from University of Hong Kong fMRI of acupuncture on 17 healthy males. The acupuncture points stimulated were TW-8 and GV-15, both of which were called "language-implicated acupoints." This may have been a reference to other research on the effect of these acupoints on the brain's language centers.[3]

Chapter 28
Anxiousness

Anxiety is a mood disorder characterized by apprehension, uncertainty, and fear that is out of proportion to any known cause. Other terms that may be used to describe this include "anxiety disorder" or "anxiety reaction". "Panic disorder" or a panic attack would also fall into the more extreme end of this category. It can often elevate to attacks of intense panic associated with bodily reactions, some symptoms may include:
-Fatigue
-Irritability
-Muscle tension
-Restlessness
-Decreased concentration
-Sleep pattern changes

When the fear comes on intensely and suddenly it is referred to as a panic attack. Panic disorder describes repeated panic attacks followed by concern over future attacks or changes in behavior related to the panic attack. Other accompanying symptoms can include:
-Heart palpitations
-Shortness of breath
-Trembling
-Feeling of choking or suffocation
-Chest pain
-Abdominal symptoms
-Dizziness
-Loss of sense of reality/dissociation
-Fear of losing control or dying
-Chills, hot flashes, or a feeling of numbness/tingling.

Due to survivors potentially experiencing slowed information processing speed, difficulty with problem solving, or difficulty concentrating, they may feel overwhelmed when faced with situations where decisions need made or a lot of things are happening at once. For this reason, parties, community outings, heavy traffic, or similar situations can induce a significant level of anxiety. Additionally, someone may have anxiety or fear over falling and sustaining further injury as a result of chronic pain. Memory impairments can induce anxiety in situations where they may forget where they are, what they are doing, or people who are around them such as caregivers or even family members.

The department of veteran affairs system found that approximately 25% of all veterans following active duty in Iraq and Afghanistan received a mental health diagnosis and 11% were found to have a form of mood disorder. One study found panic disorders occurring in a TBI population at a rate of 9.2% over 7.5 years. In genetic testing there was evidence to support that the presence of a predisposing factor to the development of psychiatric disorders after a severe TBI, apolipoprotein E epsilon 4 (APOE*E4). The interactions between genetic predisposition and environmental influences such as early childhood struggles (such as history of abuse), life stress, and limited support structures may increase risk of development of mood disorders.

Glutamate, with its role in excitotoxic injury and maladaptive stress responses, also plays a role in mood regulation through the hippocampus and prefrontal cortex. Significant shrinking of the hippocampus has been found in those who have sustained a brain injury and developed mood disorders compared to those with similar injuries but no changes in mood.

Anxiety can result from the conditions surrounding an injury, brain regions affected, damage to the neurotransmitter system, or any/all of the above. Anxiety coupled with depression tends to be in the right hemisphere, in contrast to depression only which tends to be shown in the left hemisphere.

Etiology:
Anxiety can be physiological and/or psychological. There may be a genetic tendency present. The physiologic factors involved stem around arousal of the autonomic nervous system in the manner of a "fight or flight" response to fearful inner impulses and emotions. This stress response results in the characteristic body sensations often seen in a person in a panic attack.

Psychologic factors vary with one's experience, but usually some sort of emotional stress happens before the anxiety. The emotional stress might be easily identifiable (such as the loss of a job or relationship),. It could, however, be subconscious and harder to uncover, such as when hidden inner emotional drives of neediness, sexuality, and aggression are kept out of conscious thought by psychological defenses. When these troubles are brought up by a social or environmental event that rouses the person, the feelings of anxiety can represent their fear of losing control of these repressed conflicts and, in turn, their actions.

Another reason for anxiety can be a known or subconsciously hidden trauma that certain situations or events can trigger. The person may then revert to the traumatic event, setting up the resulting fight or flight response.

Signs & Symptoms
-Severity of worry exceeds what the situation warrants
-Restlessness
-Fatigue
-Difficulty concentrating
-Irritability
-Muscle tension
-Insomnia

Diagnosis
-At least 3 of the above signs

Differential Diagnosis:
Medical Disorders:
  -Hyperthyroidism or hypothyroidism
  -Other endocrinological disorders (hyperparathyroidism, adrenal tumor etc.)
  -Cardiac arrythmias
  -Seizure disorders
  -Hypoglycemia

Effects of Substances:
>   -Alcohol abuse or or illicit substance intoxication or withrawal
>   -Medication side effects

Psychiatric Disorders:
>   -Panic disorder with or without agoraphobia
>   -Generalized Anxiety Disorder (GAD)
>   -Post-Traumatic Stress Disorder (PTSD)
>   -Obsessive-Compulsive Disorder (OCD)
>   -Social Phobia and specific phobias
>   -Schizophrenia and other psychotic disorders

Biomedical Approaches
-Benzodiazepines
-SSRI's
-Psychotherapy
-Peer support or family therapy
-Biofeedback

Natural Treatment Approaches

Dietary Considerations
Maintain an overall healthy diet – Use fresh foods as close to the natural state as possible, avoiding prepackaged and processed foods. Eat daily servings of leafy green vegetables, whole grains (such as brown rice and millet), fresh fruit, and proteins with a minimum of animal fat. Drink at least 8 cups of fluids daily.

Therapeutic foods:
- Increase foods that calm the Shen (Spirit), tonify the Heart, harmonize the Stomach and Spleen, clear Heat, invigorate the Liver Qi
- Longan, oyster, rice, rosemary, wheat, wheat germ, mushroom
- Oatmeal
- Foods high in B-complex vitamins, oysters, celery, sesame seeds, tahini, calming foods, oatstraw juice and oats, collards, kelp, cherry, cucumber, corn, grapes, chicory, apples, kale, honey, mulberry, carrot

Avoid:
- Eliminate stimulants, especially those containing caffeine: coffee, chocolate, cola, black tea
- Foods with malic acids: most apples (apples without malic acid: Astrachan, Belleflower, Jonathan, Delicious); coffee, tea, fried foods, sugar and sweet foods
- Meat, alcohol, hot sauces, spicy foods, fatty foods, rich foods, salty foods, food additives, tobacco

Somatic Therapeutic Considerations
-Meditation, guided relaxation
-QiGong/Tai Qu Chuan
-Yoga
-Exercise

Orthomolecular Considerations

-L-Theranine
-Phosphorus
-Lithium
-B vitamin complex (50mg BID)
-Calcium (1,000 mg/day, taken at bed time)
-Magnesium (500 mg/ day)
-L-tryptophan
-Omega 3 fatty acids
-A daily multivitamin and mineral supplement

Phytotherapeutic Considerations
-Kava Kava (250mg TID for daytime anxiety) -Ginkgo Biloba
-Valerian (150mg TID for daytime anxiety,   -Ginseng
for severe: 1 drop valerian oil to bath water) -Hops
-Ashwaganda (1 capsule or ½ teaspoon of   -Lemon Balm
tincture BID)   -Oats
-Bugleweed   -Passionflower
-California Poppy   -Peppermint
-Catnip   -St. John's Wort
-Chamomile   -Skullcap
-Fennel   -Verbena
-Feverfew

Acupressure/Tapping Considerations
--PC-6, HT-3, HT-8, KI-1, CV-17, Yintang, Ear Shenmen
Clinical Notes:
-Intradermal needles or ear seeds may be helpful at ear Shenmen or PC-6 to allow for
stimulation of these points between appointments. Patients may also find this personally
empowering as they can press or massage these points in the event anxious feelings arise to
aid in subduing symptoms.

-L-Theanine, an active ingredient in green tea, and available as a supplement, can be quite
useful. It can be taken either in a low dose daily for general anxiety or symptomatically as
needed. In the occurrence of panic attacks higher doses can be taken to abate symptoms.
The relative safety, positive benefits of L-theanine on the brain, and low occurrence of side
effects makes this an appealing option.

Chapter 29
Depressive Disorders

Depression is a disorder characterized by mood disturbance, psychomotor dysfunction, and vegetative symptoms. Primary when it is the first mental disorder to appear, it is considered secondary when it appears with another psychiatric or medical condition. It may also be associated with aggressive behavior

Reported prevalence of depressive disorders following a brain injury range from 6% up to a staggering 77% depending on the study and the data pool. Long term studies indicate 44% of individuals with TBI were at a much higher risk of depression within 7.5 years after an injury. Severe injuries have shown lower rates of depression than more mild injuries. This may be the result of levels of self-awareness of symptoms playing a role in reports. Major depressive disorder is very often found alongside anxiety disorder. Apathy can also co-occur.

Major depression has been shown to happen in injuries to the left dorsolateral frontal lobe, and/or left basal ganglia. Right hemisphere and parieto-occipital injuries demonstrated less severe symptoms. Diffuse axonal damage can progress over weeks or months to further impact vulnerable regions such as the neocortex, hippocampus, amygdala, thalamus, and striatum. Dreverts[1] puts forth that major depression could result from the deactivation of frontal brain regions while there is an increase in activation of the limbic and paralimbic structures, including the amygdala.

Cognitive changes in TBI survivors remain consistent with left lateral prefrontal difficulties. In athletes who have experienced a concussion and presented with depression there was a consistent finding of lowered activation of the dorsolateral prefrontal cortex and striatum as well as local grey matter loss.

A brain injury can affect modulating neural systems which can then affect mood. Depletion of serotonin transmission has been associated with emotional disturbances, disinhibition, aggressive behavior, and may play a role in depressive disorders. Changes in dopamine transmission is associated with apathy as well as affecting executive and memory functions. Deficits in the forebrain cholinergic system have been associated with behavioral changes including lack of motivation, agitation, disinhibition and anhedonia.

Etiology

Genetics
-Impaired limbic-diencephalon function
-Extrapyramidal structures
-Acetylcholine
-Norepinephrine, Dopamine
-Serotonin

Physiologic
-Chronic Pain or illness
-Chronic stress
-Hypoglycemia
-Hormonal imbalances
-Nutritional deficiencies (B6, B12, iron, Thiamin, C)

-Aspartic Acid Excess
-Asparagine Excess

Drug and alcohol abuse
Drug Reactions
-Steroids
-Digitalis
-Oral contraceptives
-Blood pressure medications
-Appetite suppressants

-Aspirin

Environmental
-Heavy metal exposure
-Industrial solvent exposure
-Toxin exposure

Personality
-Introversion
-Anxiety

Signs & Symptoms
-Depressed, irritable, anxious feelings
-Furrowed brows, slumped posture
-Monosyllabic speech
-Guilt
-Difficulty concentrating
-Indecisiveness

-Loss of interest
-Social withdrawal
-Helplessness, hopelessness
-Recurrent thoughts of death and suicide
-Inability to experience emotions
-Sleep disorders

Diagnosis
- Depressed mood
- Apathy/Loss of Interest
+
- Weight/Appetite change
- Sleep disturbances
- Psychomotor change
- Guilt/Worthlessness
- Cognitive dysfunction
- Suicidal Ideation
- Hair analysis for heavy metals

Norepinephrine/Dopamine	Serotonin
-Motivation -Energy -Interest -Concentration	-Impulsivity -Change in sexual activity -Change in appetite

Differential Diagnosis
-Adjustment disorder with depressed mood
-Frontal Lobe Syndrome
-Apathy
-Emotional lability
-PTSD

Biomedical Approaches
- SSRI's
- Heterocyclic antidepressants
- 5-HT antagonists
- Psychotherapy

Natural Treatment Approaches

Dietary Considerations
Eating principles:
-Consider food sensitivities
-Consume enough high quality protein. Replace red meat with fish and chicken as much as possible and include beans, nuts and seeds
-Hypoglycemic diet
-Treat hypothyroidism if present: Low thyroid function is a very common cause of depression.
-Chelate heavy metals if present
-Avoid toxic fumes including cigarette smoke. Inhaling toxic fumes results in an increased level of cortisol and may exacerbate a pre-existing hypoglycemia. Cortisol decreases the uptake of tryptophan in the brain resulting in decreased levels of serotonin.
-Elimination/rotation diet, rotation diet, rotation diet expanded

Therapeutic foods:
-Foods high in omega-3 fatty acids: nut, seed, vegetable oils (safflower, canola, walnut, sunflower, flax seed), evening primrose oil, black currant oil
-Foods rich in Vitamin B6
-Foods high in tryptophan: nuts, eggs, meat, fish, dairy
-If supplementing tryptophan: include cofactors (Vitamins B3, B6, and C) and whole wheat toast, bananas, walnuts, pineapples that are high in serotonin

Specific foods
Stagnant Liver Qi or Stagnancy in the Liver channel:
-Citrus peel, figs, honey
-Liver-cleansing foods: beets, carrots, artichokes, lemons, parsnips, dandelion greens, watercress, burdock root

Avoid:
- Hypoglycemia
- Foods containing tyramine if the patient is on MAO inhibitors. Cheese, chicken, liver, sardines, red wine, yeast, beer, soured cream, eggplant, and green bean pods should all be avoided.
- Aspartame which increases CNS tyrosine and phenylalanine while decreasing tryptophan availability. This results in decreased levels of serotonin in the brain.
- Consider food sensitivities, avoid food intolerances
- Meat, alcohol, hot sauces, spicy foods, fried foods, fatty foods, rich foods, salty foods
- Coffee, caffeine
- Sugar, diet high in simple carbohydrates, especially if indications of hypoglycemia.

Somatic Therapy Considerations
-Exercise is of tremendous benefit in improving one's mental health. At least 30 minutes 3 times per week should be engaged in physical exercise that will get the heart working vigorously such as brisk walking, aerobics, swimming, etc.
-Meditation
-Qigong, Tai Qi Chuan

-Light Therapy

Orthomolecular Considerations
- B vitamins (particularly B12)
- Amino acids
- Tryptophan
- Tyrosine
- Phenylalanine
- L-Theanine
- DHEA
- SAMe
- 5-HTP
-Magnesium
-Lithium
-Selenium
-Omega-3

Phytotherapeutic Considerations:

- St. John's Wort (300mg TID)
- Kava-Kava (400-600 mg BID)
- Lemon Balm leaves (1 to 2 cups of tea per day for 1 to 2 weeks)
- Cayenne Pepper (1/4 teaspoon TID, encapsulation may improve compliance)
- Ginkgo Biloba
- Licorice
- Siberian Ginseng
- Damiana
- Basil
- Black Hellebore
- Borage
- Clove
- Ginger
- Oat Straw Purslane
- Rosemary
- Sage
- Thyme
- Yohimbine
- He Shou Wu (Fo Ti)
- Culver's Root
-Valerian

Acupressure/Tapping Considerations
ST-36, LR-3, LR-14, GV-20, GV-24

Acupuncture Research Studies:
-A multi-centered collaborative study was conducted, in which 241 inpatients with depression were recruited. Patients were randomly divided into two treatment groups: electro-acupuncture (EA) + placebo and a amitriptyline group. The results showed that the therapeutic efficacy of EA was equal to that of amitriptyline for depressive disorders ($P > 0.05$). Electro-acupuncture had a better therapeutic effect for anxiety somatization and cognitive process disturbance of depressed patients than amitriptyline ($P < 0.05$). Moreover, the side effects of EA were much less than that of amitriptyline ($P < 0.001$).[3]

-A meta-analysis of post-stroke depression reviewed 15 studies of 1096 patients. Comparison between the acupuncture group and Western medicine group concluded a statistical difference in curative rate and remarkably effective rate, but no difference in effective rate.[4]

-Researchers from Jinan University (Guangzhou, China) conclude that acupuncture is effective for the alleviation of depression. In the study, the acupuncture treatment group achieved a total efficacy rate of 88.9% and the drug control group achieved an efficacy rate of 84.8%. Patients in the control group received administration of the pharmaceutical medication fluoxetine (Prozac). The researchers conclude that acupuncture slightly outperforms fluoxetine for the treatment of depression. In addition, acupuncture treatment displays certain advantages compared with anti-depressant drugs. Acupuncture achieved a higher cure rate and the drugs had a significant adverse reaction rate. [5]

- After being exposed to a chronic unpredicted stress procedure for 2 weeks, rats were subjected to electro-acupuncture (EA) treatment, which was performed on acupoints GV-20 and GB-34, once every other day for 15 consecutive days (including 8 treatments), with each treatment lasting for 30 min. The behavioural tests (i.e., forced swimming test, elevated plus-maze test, and open-field entries test) revealed that EA alleviated the depressive-like and anxiety-like behaviours of the stressed rats. Immunohistochemical results showed that proliferative cells (BrdU-positive) in the EA group were significantly larger in number compared with the Model group. Further, the results showed that EA significantly promoted the proliferation of amplifying neural progenitors (ANPs) and simultaneously inhibited the apoptosis of quiescent neural progenitors (QNPs). [2]

-Electrical acupuncture has been found in clinical studies to be effective for the treatment of depression: GV-20 and GV-24 OR GV-20 and Yin Tang. Set at 2Hz continuous frequency; if anxiety is present with depression, set at 2/100 Hz mixed frequency

Chapter 30
Mania

A manic episode is when an individual has a markedly elevated, expansive, or irritable mood for at least one week along with at least three of the following symptoms:
-Extremely amplified self-esteem
-Decreased desire for sleep
-Grandiose ideation
-Distractability
-High-risk behaviors

Individuals may experience
-Hyperactivity
-Distractabillity, Flightiness of ideas
-Hypersexuality, disinhibited sexuality
-Tangentality
-Delusions, usually of grandeur
-Confabulation
-Indiscriminant financial activity or irresponsibility
-Decreased need for sleep
-Pressured Speech
-Emotional lability
-Increased aggression

While laughing and joking one moment, individuals may quickly become irritated, angered, enraged, destructive, or conversely tearful and depressed with slight provocation. That is, manic-depressive symptoms can occur (explored in the next chapter), with mania being dominant. Hence, bipolar affective disturbances can be due to waxing and waning abnormalities involving the right and left frontal lobes.

Relation to brain injury:
It has been theorized that mania may relate to temporal pole injuries and multi-location injuries. This seems to be a more defining factor than the severity of the injury or other factors like family history or social factors. Increased aggression with a lessened euphoria may point to mania as a result of a brain injury rather than those stemming from other causes.

Differential Diagnosis
-Substance-induced mood disorder
-Psychosis associated with epilepsy
-Personality change as a result of brain injury

Biomedical Treatment
Lithium carbonate
Anticonvulsants
       -Carbamazepine (Tegretol)
       -Valproate (Depakote)
       -Lamotrigine (Lamictal)
       -Topiramate (Topamax)
       -Clonazepam (Klonopin)
Antipsychotics
       -Olanzapine (Zyprexa)
       -Quetiapine (Seroquel

-Risperidone (Risperdal)
-Aripiprazole (Abilify)
Verapamil (calcium channel blocker)
Benzodiazepines (short course)
Psychotherapy

Natural Treatment Approaches

Classical Treatments:[5, 6]
Diankuang caused by the one hundred pathologic factors: 13 Ghost Points – Sun Simiao
Kuang – one jumps and runs: CV-13, HT-7
Attack of kuang: HT-3, PC-5, LI-11, SI-3, GB-1, KI-7
Hyperexcitation: ST-45, St-42
Sudden hyperexcitation, hallucinations, violent sweats: PC-5
Attacks of hyperexcitation: HT-3, BL-43, CV-14, LR-8, CV-13, HT-7
Overexcitation from emotional agitation: GB-35, BL-18
Prolonged hyperexcitation, climbs up, sings, takes off clothes, runs: ST-45, ST-42, ST-40
Hyperexcitation becomes apoplexy (Stroke): GB-39

Auricular Points:
Shenmen, Point Zero, Sympathetic, Heart, Liver, Apex

Clinical Notes:
- Patients exhibiting manic symptoms may have difficulty lying still long enough to perform a full body treatment. They may be verbose and flighty in both mind and bodily movements. It is possible that they may even remove needles that have been inserted, wanting to move and finding the increased sensation irritating. Auricular points may be helpful in an attempt to calm them quickly and possibly allow for a fuller treatment. Yintang or bleeding ear apex may also be helpful in this regard. Ear seeds may be helpful between treatments if the patient will keep them in.

Acupressure/Tapping Considerations
PC-5, GV-26, Ear Apex, HT-8, HT-9, Yintang, Ear Shenmen
-Massage at KI-1 may also be considered to help ground the patient and promote an inward and downward movement of Qi

Chapter 31
Bipolar Disorder

Bipolar Affective Disorder (BAD) is characterized by mood disturbance that involve periods of abnormally elevated mood (mania) and abnormally low mood (depression), motor dysfunction, and autonomic symptoms. It affects 5% of the population and affects genders equally, though females tend to have depressive forms more often while males tend to more frequently have manic forms. In 85% of cases, depression dominates the personality cycle.

Bipolar disorder is associated with an enhanced sensitivity to dopamine, increased norepinephrine, serotonin, and dopamine production, and an upregulation of glutamate. As discussed in the chapter on anxiety disorders, each of these neurotransmitter channels can be affected by a brain injury. Due to the heightened dopamine sensitivity, bipolar has also shown links to schizophrenic disorders.

There have been noted increases in white matter abnormalities, which tend to happen with demyelination, glial cell inflammation, axonal loss, or aging brains. The prefrontal cortex and hippocampus have been shown to have lower grey matter volume (as much as 25-40%) in people with BAD. Changes showing shrinkage of the cerebellum can also occur, which can limit communication between the limbic and frontal regions. Lowered glucose and blood flow use have also been shown.

Subtypes
Bipolar I – one or more manic episodes with a preceding hypomanic stage
Bipolar II – one or more depressive episodes followed by one or more hypomanic episodes without full mania
Cyclothymic disorder - chronic fluctuating mood disturbance with both depressive and hypomanic states

Etiology
-Brain Injury
-Genetics
-Stressors
-Personality - extroverted, achievement oriented

Signs & Symptoms
-Sudden onset
-Shorter cycles than unipolar depression - 3-6 months
-Depressive symptoms similar to unipolar depression
-Lessened motor movement
-Excessive sleeping

Signs of manic psychosis
-Elation	-Extreme activity	-Racing thoughts
-Irritability	-Lack of insight	-Distractable
-Hostility	-Believe they are at their best	-Delusional grandiosity
-Rapid speech	-Paranoid delusions	-Auditory and visual

hallucinations   -Need less sleep
                                    -Inexhaustible, impulsive

Diagnosic Testing
-Ultrasound of the head
-CAT scan
-EEG
-Full Blood Count
-Thyroid and liver function tests
-Urine and creatine levels assessment

Biomedical Treatment
Lithium carbonate 300 mg 2-5x/day, 0.3-0.8 mEq/L maintenance
            many side effects: tremor, muscle spasms, nausea, vomiting, diarrhea, thirst ,
            polydipsia, polyuria, acne, psoriasis, hypothyroidism, nephrogenic diabetes,
            confusion, seizures, arrhythmia. flaxseed oil helps decrease side effects (1-3
            tbsp/day)
Anticonvulsants
            -Carbamazepine (Tegretol)
            -Valproate (Depakote)
            -Lamotrigine (Lamictal)
            -Topiramate (Topamax)
Antipsychotics
            -Olanzapine (Zyprexa)
Benzodiazepines (short course)
Psychotherapy

Possible Co-morbidities
-Head trauma
-Substance abuse
-PTSD-Obsessive Compulsive Disorder
-Eating disorders

Natural Treatment Approaches

Dietary Considerations:
Therapeutic foods:
-Increase foods rich in Vitamin B-complex and Vitamin C
-Longan, oyster, rice, rosemary, wheat, wheat germ, mushroom
-Sour foods,
-Dispersing foods, foods that open channels - citrus peel, figs, honey
-Liver-cleansing foods: beets, carrots, artichokes, lemons, parsnips, dandelion greens,
watercress, burdock root
-Vitamin C foods

Avoid:
- Meat, alcohol, hot sauces, spicy foods, fried foods, fatty foods, rich foods, salty foods,
coffee, caffeine, sweet foods and sugar

Somatic Therapy Considerations:
- Qigong
- Tai qi chuan
-Meditation/mindfullness practice

Orthomolecular Considerations
- EPA/DHA greatly stabilizes mood stopping rapid mood cycling.
- Lecithin (phosphatidylcholine) (15-30gm) to prevent mania
- Vitamin C
- Vitamin E
- B Vitamins
- L-tryptophan is helpful in some studies, others not. High doses used – caused nausea.
- 5-HTP has helped (50%) but can cause increase in serotonin inducing mania
-N-Acetyl Cysteine
- Multi-vitamin

Phytotherapeutic Considerations
-St. John's Wort
-Skullcap
-Valerian
-Siberian Ginseng

Acupressure/Tapping Considerations
According to either Depressive phase (chapter 29) or Manic phase (chapter 30)

Chapter 32
Post-Traumatic Stress Disorder (PTSD)

The after effect of a highly stressful situation can cause a chronic cluster of emotional and physical symptoms where someone re-experiences the traumatic event. This causes intense fear, helplessness, and avoidance of stimulation associated with the trauma. PTSD awareness has seen an upsurge in recent decades and its connections to brain injuries within military personnel, and community or mass traumas.

In the United States an estimated 7-9% of the population are affected by PTSD. This rate increases in populations with a higher risk of repeated exposure to traumatic events such as paramedics, firefighters, etc. which ranges from 17-22%. If someone has sustained a head injury, from an automobile accident or some other cause, percentages ranged from 13-33% developing some degree of PTSD. Military personnel are estimated to range in rates from 10-30% with combat exposure increasing the risk and being a major factor even when compared to deployment without combat exposure. Because of the increase in blast injuries, head injuries and PTSD are becoming more and more frequently found together. It has been reported in a 2008 study that 43.9% of military personnel who reported a TBI with loss of consciousness met criteria for PTSD.

PTSD acts as a continuation and magnification of anxiety-related symptoms which fit into three primary symptom clusters – reexperiencing, avoidance, and hyperarousal. For a diagnosis these symptoms need to be present for at least one month and impair the individual's ability to function in a social, occupational or other important life arena.

Diagnostic criteria for PTSD	
Activity	**Possible Symptoms**
Exposure to or witnessing of a threatening event	Intense fear Helplessness Horror Symptoms of reexperiencing
Recurrent or intrusive memories	Nightmares Sense of reliving the trauma Psychological or physical distress when reminded of the trauma
Avoidance	Inability to recall parts of the trauma Withdrawal Emotional numbing
Increased autonomic arousal	Sleep disturbances Irritability Hypervigilance Difficulty concentrating Exaggerated startle response

Factors in the development of PTSD	
Pre-traumatic factors	-Ongoing life stress or demographics -Lack of social support -Young age at time of trauma -Pre-existing psychiatric disorder -Low socio-economic status, education level, intelligence, -Prior trauma exposure (reported abuse in childhood, report of other previous trauma, report of other adverse childhood factors -Family history of psychiatric disorders
Peri-traumatic or trauma related factors	-Severe trauma -Type of trauma (interpesonal traumas such as torture, rape or assault convey a high risk of PTSD) -High perceived threat to life -Community (mass) trauma -Peritraumatic dissociation
Post-traumatic factors	-Ongoing life stress -Lack of positive social support -Negative social support (ex: negative reactions from others) -Bereavement -Major loss of resources -Other factors, including children at home and distressed spouse

Many symptoms that present with PTSD are similar to or can also found in brain injuries such as cognitive impairments (poor attention and memory), behavioral components (impulsivity, disinhibition) and emotional changes (emotional lability, depression). Secondary effects such as social isolation, difficulty in interpersonal relations, and difficulties functioning in home and work environments may also become problematic. Due to these similarities, it is possible that they have similar or the same brain regions and functions affected in both.

When both are present it has been suggested that a brain injury can make it more difficult to cope with the stress of PTSD through disinhibition of executive function while PTSD can affect the cognitive problems that can follow a brain injury. As a result, this interplay can be difficult for an individual to manage.

Comparison of symptoms between PTSD and brain injury		
PTSD	Found in both PTSD and Brain Injury	Brain Injury
Flashbacks Avoidance Hypervigilance Nightmares Reexperiencing	Fatigue Irritability Insomnia Depression Cognitive deficits	Headache Nausea/vomiting Photophobia or noise sensitivity Vision problems

216

Brain regions often affected by PTSD tend to overlap with those also most often affected by a brain injury. Among these are:
-Medial prefrontal cortex
-Anterior cingulate cortex
-Temporal region
-Hippocampus
-Amygdala.

It has been suggested that PTSD is characterized by an overactive amygdala along with an underactive medial prefrontal cortex. Here the prefrontal cortex fails to subdue the heightened fear reactions of the amygdala. Executive function impairment can also increase the tenacity of the re-experiencing effect. The hippocampus has also been shown to atrophy and shrink in size in PTSD. This shrinking does not occur within the first six months post-injury, but rather a while after the event and does not seem to occur in children.

Serotonin pathways seem to be affected by PTSD, as such, SSRI drugs have often been used for PTSD symptoms as benefits has been demonstrated. These SSRIs also change release of norepinephrine, which directly impacts startle response, the prefrontal cortex inhibition of the amygdala, and recollection of the traumatic event, all of which create a feedback loop of memory consolidation. GABA has also been demonstrated to be lessened while the excitatory neurotransmitter, glutamate, increased. Acetylcholine regulation may also be impacted and have cognitive effects.

Hormonal changes associated with PTSD show a tendency to have low levels of the stress hormone cortisol high levels of corticotropin-releasing factor (CRF). Typically with a response to stress there are high levels of CRF and cortisol. This difference was originally thought to be due to adrenal fatigue, but emergency room studies showed low to normal levels of cortisol as well. It has since been shown that those with PTSD have increased numbers of cortisol receptors and that these have an increased sensitivity. This allows for greater bodily control over the cortisol that is released.

It has been proposed that post-injury amnesia, particularly in severe brain injuries, may actually act as a "protective mechanism" against the development of PTSD as most cases with severe TBI do not meet criteria for PTSD. It is the mild cases of brain injury that seem to demonstrate the highest rates of PTSD development.

Etiology:
Although a traumatic event is the trigger for the anxiety disorder known as PTSD, not all people experiencing traumatic events acquire the continued acute emotional responses to it.

Another factor in the development of PTSD, outside of the traumatic event, is the person's own innate ability to process and cope with the stress. While some soldiers become "battle-fatigued" following combat, others emerge from battle exhilarated by the encounter. It is hard to determine who exactly is at highest risk for development of PTSD in situations of severe stress (like soldiers before going to battle, or survivors of a massive natural disaster). Perceived mental or physical tenacity or strength have little bearing in the face of severely traumatic events. Anyone, no matter their degree of training or preparation, can develop PTSD. Others who may be suspected to handle stress poorly may seem relatively unaffected in the long term by such experiences. This is likely due to the numerous factors beyond fortitude of the mind that have been discussed in this chapter, many of which are neurobiologically set. For this reason, all who encounter significant stressors should be mindful of or made aware of any personality, emotional or physical changes that might signify the beginnings of PTSD.

Signs & Symptoms
-Re-experience of some traumatic event:
        -nightmares
        -flashbacks
-Persistent avoidance of stimuli
-Increased arousal
-Anger or irritability
-Depression

Types of stressors that can induce PTSD:
- Threat to one's life or physical integrity
- Serious threat or harm to one's children, spouse, other close relatives, or friends
- Destruction of one's home or community
- Seeing another person who is mutilated, dying, or dead
- Being the victim of physical violence (including child abuse)

Biomedical Approaches
Anti Depressants (SSRI's)
        -Fluoxetine
        -Sertaline
        -Partoxetine
Mood Stabilizers – Lamotrigine
Atypical antipsychotics – Olanzapine
Beta-blockers - Propanalol
Psychotherapy
        -Cognitive-behavioral (individual and group, trauma-focused or traditional)
        -Exposure Therapy
        -Stress management

Natural Treatment Approaches
Dietary Considerations:
Therapeutic foods:
- Increase foods that calm the Shen, tonify the Heart, harmonize the Stomach and Spleen

Avoid:
- Meat, alcohol, hot sauces, spicy foods, fried foods, fatty foods, rich foods, salty foods, coffee, caffeine, sweet foods and sugar

Somatic Therapy Considerations:
- Aerobic exercise: regular exercise helps minimize stress
- Qigong
- Tai Qi Chuan
-Trauma Release Exercises (TRE)
-Eye Movement Desensitization and Reprocessing (EMDR)

218

-Body-based psychotherapies (Bioenergetics, Reichian therapy, Hakomi, Core Energetics, etc)

Orthomolecular Considerations

Recommended micronutrient preparation for PTSD by Dr. Prasad	
Vitamin A	3,000 IU
Natural Vitamin E	400 IU
Vitamin C	1,000 mg
Vitamin D3	1,000 IU
Vitamin B1	10 mg
Vitamin B2	4 mg
Vitamin B3	100 mg
Vitamin B6	4 mg
Folic Acid	400 mcg
Vitamin B12	100 mcg
Biotin	150 mcg
Pantothenic Acid	15 mg
Zinc glycinate	5 mg
Selenium	100 mcg
N-acetylcyateine	Proprietary amount
Coenzyme Q10	Proprietary amount
Alpha-lipoic Acid	Proprietary amount
L-Carnitine	Proprietary amount
Resveratrol	Proprietary amount
Curcumin	Proprietary amount
Omega-3 Fatty Acids	Proprietary amount

Phytotherapeutic Considerations
-Panax Ginselng
-Valerian
-Sumbul
-Curcumin
-Hops
-Wild Oats
-Passionflower
-Skullcap

219

Acupuncture Research Studies:

- A systematic review synthesized evidence from seven studies which met criteria with 709 total participants included. Studies compared acupuncture with treatment as usual (TAU), sham acupuncture, a passive waitlist control, cognitive behavioral therapy, and paroxetine. Statistically significant effects in favor of acupuncture (as adjunctive or monotherapy) were found versus any comparator for PTSD symptoms at postintervention. Safety data suggested that acupuncture is not associated with any serious adverse events. No systematic differences by type of acupuncture were found in those comparingsuch data. Potential benefits of acupuncture for PTSD and depression symptoms were identified compared with control groups in the months following treatment.[5]

-Fifty-five service members meeting research diagnostic criteria for PTSD were randomized to usual PTSD care (UPC) plus eight 60-minute sessions of acupuncture conducted twice weekly or to UPC alone. Outcomes were assessed at baseline and 4, 8, and 12 weeks post-randomization. It was found that Mean improvement in PTSD severity was significantly greater among those receiving acupuncture than in those receiving UPC. Acupuncture was also associated with significantly greater improvements in depression, pain, and physical and mental health functioning. The study concluded acupuncture being effective for reducing PTSD symptoms.[6]

-138 patients with earthquake-caused PTSD who enrolled were randomly assigned to an electro-acupuncture group and an oral paroxetine group. The electro-acupuncture group was treated by scalp electro-acupuncture on Baihui (GV 20), Sishencong (EX-HN 1), Shenting (GV 24), and Fengchi (GB 20). The efficacy and safety of the electro-acupuncture on treatment of 69 PTSD patients were evaluated using Clinician-Administered PTSD Scale (CAPS), Hamilton Depression Scale (HAMD), Hamilton Anxiety Scale (HAMA), and Treatment Emergent Symptom Scale (TESS). Efficacy in the electro-acupuncture group was found significantly better than that in the paroxetine group.[7]

-A systematic review of randomized control trials showed "One high-quality RCT reported that acupuncture was superior to wait list control and therapeutic effects of acupuncture and cognitive-behavioral therapy (CBT) were similar based on the effect sizes. One RCT showed no statistical difference between acupuncture and selective serotonin reuptake inhibitors (SSRIs). One RCT reported a favorable effect of acupoint stimulation plus CBT against CBT alone. A meta-analysis of acupuncture plus moxibustion versus SSRI favored acupuncture plus moxibustion in three outcomes." suggesting "that the evidence of effectiveness of acupuncture for PTSD is encouraging".[8]

-Journal of mental and Nervous Diseases published a study evaluating the possible efficacy and acceptability of acupuncture for posttraumatic stress disorder (PTSD). People diagnosed with PTSD were randomized to either an empirically developed acupuncture treatment (ACU), a group cognitive-behavioral therapy (CBT), or a wait-list control (WLC). The primary outcome measure was self-reported PTSD symptoms at baseline, end treatment, and 3-month follow-up. Compared with the wait list group, acupuncture provided large treatment effects for PTSD similar in magnitude to the cognitive behavioral group. Symptom reductions at end treatment were maintained at 3-month follow-up for both interventions. [9]

Chapter 33
Behavioral Changes and Emotional Lability

Behavioral changes can often be a problematic sequelae of a brain injury impacting one's social interactions with family, friends, support systems, employers and others. This may be to the degree of losing these relationships all together. This results in a sense of loneliness or isolation. At times they may result in further consequences such as substance abuse, incarceration, homelessness, psychiatric hospitalization, and victimization.

These changes may be temporary or last a lifetime. Many individuals coming out of a coma display a period of increased irritability, confusion, physical restlessness, disorientation and confabulation. Some individuals will develop a quick temper following their injury in which they often yell, curse, hit, kick, and throw things. These can be triggered by feelings of frustration, being misunderstood, isolation, or difficulty in concentration. These have been suspected to be pre-injury traits or tendencies that are exacerbated in the face of being overstimulated. Some will involuntarily express of the opposite emotion of that which they are actually feeling such as laughing when they are in fact sad. This can cause a lot of difficulty in their interactions with others and frustration for all involved. A pseudobulbar effect, also known as emotional incontinence, can develop in which emotions spontaneous arise without any particular event or trigger.

Common Neurobehavioral Complications of Brain Injury		
-Aggression	-Eating Disturbances	-Poor judgment and reasoning
-Agitation/irritability	-Flat affect/restricted	-Dysphoria
-Apathy	emotions	-Delusions
-Denial of deficits	-Inability to recognize	-Euphoria
-Childish behavior	emotions	-Aberrant movements
-Poor self-awareness	-Impulsivity	-Psychosis (rare)
-Loss of sense of self	-Lability/emotional instability	
-Disinhibition	-Poor initiation	

Lezak described five primary personality changes that can occur after a TBI:
-Impaired social perceptiveness
-Impaired self control and regulation
-Stimulus bound behavior
-Emotional change
-Inability to learn from personal experience

Brain-based reasons for such changes is dependent on the site of injury and the extent of damage done. Diffuse axonal injuries may result in an "unplugging" of the neural networks from one another and less interaction with the remainder of the CNS during functional activities. The vetromedial prefrontal cortex mediates between emotional and moral cognition. Moral judgment is associated with activation of the right temporal cortex, lenticular nucleus, and the cerebellum; whereas judgments not containing emotional significance showed activation of the frontal polar cortex and medial frontal gyrus.

221

Reactions and psychological defenses in response to noxious stimuli stems from an interaction between limbic drives, paralimbic cortical inhibition, and contextual relations tied to past events/experiences. Some individuals find that they are much more driven toward sensation-seeking behaviors. That is, they become "adrenaline junkies" - seeking out activities that provide a "rush". This is neurophysiologically linked to frontal activity. Orbitofrontal injuries often demonstrate behavioral changes such as impulsivity, euphoria, manic symptoms, and pseudobulbar effect as mentioned earlier. Specific traits have been researched and documented to relate to particular brain regions that are lined out in the table below.

Chemically, it has been suspected that dopamine receptor activity may relate to vigilance, expectation and reward. The serotonin circuits have been implicated in hostility relating to those with a type A personality type. There has also been a shown connection between high levels of catecholamines and their metabolites with better post-TBI outcomes. Many neurotransmitters are involved in aggressive behavior including norepinephrine, dopamine, acetylcholine, and GABA. Norepinephrine enhances aggressive behavior, as can elevated levels of dopamine and acetylcholine. Lowered levels of seritonergic activity and GABA, being inhibitory neurotransmitters are associated with increased aggression, or rather, disinhibition of aggressive impulses.

Brain Regions Associated with Personality Traits	
Trait	Association
Aggression	Reduced cingulate cortex volume and activity
Conditioned memory storage	Cerebellum
Decision values	Central orbitofrontal activation
Dispassionate analysis	Increased anterior cingulate activity
Emotional bias in moral decisions	Ventromedial and orbitofrontal prefrontal cortices activation
Emotional memory storage	Amygdala
Empathy/self-reflection	Insula activation
Extroversion	Reduced dorsolateral prefrontal cortex, anterior cingulate, and thalamus activity
Goal values	Medial orbitofrontal activation
Insightful/"eureka" moments	Increased superior temporal gyrus activity
Mistrust/disbelief	Reduced insula activity
Novelty seeking	Increased hippocampus and striatum activity
Optimism	Increased amygdala and anterior cingulate activity
Personal awareness of mental state	Medial prefrontal cortex
Personal space boundaries	Motor, somatosensory, cingulate and parietal cortices
Prediction errors	Ventral striatum (caudate-putamen) activation
Punctuality/subjective time sense	Substania nigra, basal ganglia and prefrontal circuits
Reflective/Comparing	Lateral prefrontal cortex activation
Self-monitoring/guiding behavior	Cingulate cortex
Social avoidance/fear/anxiety	Increased amygdala activity
Social comfort/safety	Increased striatal activity
Trust/belief	Increased ventromedial prefrontal cortex activity
Perceived unfairness	Increased insula activity

The extent to which these behavioral changes or difficulties happen depends on a number of factors including severity of the injury, personality characteristics prior to the injury, learning style, intelligence and influences of one's current environment. These environmental factors may include level of stimulation, familiarity with who they are interacting, availability of support, and demands on the individual.

Possible Methods of Controlling Environmental Factors
-Reducing noise and other extraneous stimuli -Limit visitor numbers and time -Eliminating TV and technology -Incorporate familiar objects -Repeat routines for familiarity -Provide a sense of safety (veiled beds, blankets, soft lap belts, padded hand mitts, etc)

Behavior Assessment Methods
Indirect
-Interviews
-Checklists

Direct – Direct observation of the individual
-Functional analysis/assessment
        -Minnesota Multiphasic Personality Inventory (MMPI)
        -Millon Clinical Multiaxial Inventory
        -Personality Assessment Inventory
        -Millon Behavioral Health Inventory
        -Millon Behavioral Medicine Diagnostic
-Four term contingency

Variables In Measuring Behavior		
Name	Measure	Considerations
Frequency	Count how many times a behavior occurs	Best for behaviors with a distinct start and end (striking, attending a group, asks for assistance, etc)
Rate	Point per unit of time	Can help bring perspective to frequency (10x/hour vs. 10x/week)
Duration	How long behavior lasts from start to end	e.g yelling, hand-washing, etc.
Latency	Time between stimulus and response	e.g time between a verbal cue and initiation of action
Percent Correct	Number of correct responses out of total possible number of responses	e.g number of times one correctly completes a task vs. how many total attempts

Differential Diagnosis
-Pre-injury drug and substance abuse
-Coexisting anxiety and depressive disorders
-Drug effects and side effects
       -Alcohol, cocaine, amphetamines
       -Stimulating anti-depressants
       -Antipsychotics
       -Anticholinergic medications
-Epilepsy (ictal, postictal, and interictal)
-Alzheimer's Disease
-Delirium (hypoxia, electrolyte imbalance, anesthesia and surgery, uremia, etc.)
-Infectious disease (encephalits, meningitis, pneumonia, UTI)
-Metabolic disorders (hyperthyroidism. hypothyroid, hypoglycemia, vitamin deficiency)

Biomedical Approaches
-Counseling/verbal therapies
-Use of a notebook/compensatory device
-Reinforcement protocols and behavioral treatments

Aggression
-Antipsychotics: Olanzapine, Haloperidol
-Sedatives/hypnotics: benzodiazepines – may rarely cause increased hostility, aggression, or rage
-Anti-anxiety: Buspirone, Clonazepam
-Anti-convulsants: Carbamazepine, oxcarbazepine
-Anti-manic: Lithium
-Anti-depressants: Trazadone, Sertaline, Fluoxetine
-Stimulants: Amantadine, methylphenidate
-Anti-hypertensives: Propranolol, Nadolol, Pindolol

Possible Teaching Methods for Procedures Learning	
Task Analysis	List of very specific steps involved in completing a task. Breaks larger tasks into smaller components
Shaping	Reinforcing actions that loosely resemble target behavior and easier to display by the individual
Prompting and Cueing	Individual is supported to display a correct response. These may be visual, audible, or tactile prompts
Fading	Individual learns to produce the same response under gradually changing conditions with less support over time
Generalization	Individual begins to respond similarly to different stimuli or situations they have not been trained in
Discrimination	Individual responds differently to similar stimuli based on situation

De-escalation Techniques When Working With Behavioral Disorders

224

These techniques may be helpful in situations that become very emotional, tense, or even hostile while working or interacting with an individual.

Active Listening – Good eye contact, paraphrasing, restating, clarification

Orientation – To person, place, time and purpose of activity

Redirection – Decreasing the stress of the task at hand; moving to a known or preferred skill

Setting Limits – Remaining calm; outlining all expectations and clearly defining consequences, both positive and negative outcomes stating positive outcomes first

Withdrawing Attention – Ignoring off-task behavior; helping the individual realize the relationship between attention and calm interactive behavior

Contracting – Clearly defining the parameters of expectation

Natural Approaches

Lifestyle considerations

Difficulties with control
Obsessive pondering of single ideas or thoughts, inappropriate comments, loss of inhibition, bad judgment, acts irrespective of consequences
-Quietly move the discussion forward
-Clearly respond and explain inappropriate behavior or comments
-Discuss the consequences of possible behavior or comments
-Slow down the process

Difficulties with self-awareness
Underestimation of physical or cognitive impairments, lack of insight about the condition or consequences thereof
-Provide honest feedback
-Assume the survivor ma not be entirely aware of the parameters of their symptoms

Social
Misunderstanding of social boundaries, difficulty fitting in at social events, inappropriate reactions and comments, impulsive behavior
-Establish signals to warn the person when they are overstepping
-Brief them before participating in a new social activity
-Provide constant feedback during an event to stay on track
-Carefully analyze and discuss inappropriate behavior afterward

Chapter 34
Substance Abuse

Substance abuse, both pre- and post-injury, is a very serious factor that needs assessment and appropriate treatment. In the United States alcoholism is estimated to affect 15% of the general population, while drug addiction ranges from 9-20%. In medical populations substance abuse numbers increase to between 25-50%, while those with psychiatric disorders climb to an incredible 50-75%. Treatment populations are primarily male, making up 75% . Average ages for treatment is 30-35 years in males and 25-30 years in females.

Two thirds of TBIs involve motor vehicle accidents. 50% of fatal motor vehicle accidents in the United States are associated with drugs or alcohol. Individuals with a brain injury may become addicted to medications such as opioids or turn to illegal drugs/alcohol as a means of self medicating or attempting to deal with feelings of depression, anxiety, or social isolation. A history of substance abuse has been associated with poorer healing outcomes, greater likelihood of repeat injuries, and higher risk of health deterioration later in life.[3]

Frequent complications that may arise include:
-Drug-drug interactions
-Drug overdose
-Increased sensitivity to medication effects
-Increased seizure risk.

Cognitive and emotional aspects may also be affected including:
-Increased lack of behavioral control
-Hallucinations
-Delusions
-Anxiety
-Depression.
This is especially true in relation to drug seeking or withdrawal symptoms.

Alcohol and other depressant drugs can cause depression, suicidal and homicidal thinking during intoxication. Anxiety, hyperactivity, hallucinations, and/or delusions can arise during withdrawal. Stimulant drugs can cause anxiety, hallucinations, and delusions during intoxication while possibly bringing about severe depression during withdrawal.

The compounded effects of a brain injury and substance abuse can often be additive in nature, causing significantly greater detriment. Changes in blood flow, blood-brain barrier disruption, and changes in homeostatsis are additional factors when intoxicated at the time of injury. Those hospitalized due to a brain injury and who are alcohol or drug users tend to have a longer period of hospitalization. Symptoms of agitation also tend to last longer. It is also possible that cognitive deficits such as in attention, concentration, short-term memory, and information processing speed may be further adversely affected.

Tobacco smoking prevents the immune system from working properly and increases susceptibility to disease. Cigarette smoking has been associated with worsening depression, high blood pressure, osteoporosis, arthritis, and heart disease. Withdrawal from nicotine includes symptoms such as restlessness, constipation, sweating, headaches, irritability, hunger, and inability to concentrate. Chronic nicotine use is associated with degeneration of one half of the fasciculus retroflexus which affects emotional control, sexual arousal, REM sleep, and seizure activity.[5] Smokers who have sustained a mild brain injury have been shown to have less improvement in processing speed, visual learning and memory, visuospatial skills and overall cognition compared to non-smokers.[6]

Chronic exposure to alcohol or drugs have shown changes in limbic pathways. Balanced bodily states seem to be affected in which a new biological set point, known as alleostasis, can be responsible for intense cravings. Alcohol induced atrophy of the limbic, cerebellar, and frontal structures have been shown through neuroimaging. Those with a combination of both brain injury and substance dependence showed greater degrees of shrinking than each condition on their own. GABA may be downregulated while N-methyl-D-aspartate may be upregulated due to chronic alcohol exposure.

Biomedical Approaches
-Benzodiazepines – those with short half life like lorazepam (alchohol, sedative withdrawal)
-Opioid agonists ("anti-craving"): Naltrexone, Acamprosate (alcohol)
-Disulfiram (alcohol – causes distressing side effects when alcohol is consumed including nauseau, vomiting, and headache)
-Diazepam (benzodiazepine withdrawal)
-Phenobarbital (sedative withdrawal)
-Clonidine (opiates)
-Methadone (opiates)
-Abstinence
-Confrontation of denial
-Support groups/12 step programs (e.g. alchoholics anonymous, narcotics anonymous)
-Group therapy

Note: Individuals with a brain injury seem to have reduced tolerances and increased sensitivity to a wide variety of medications, particularly sedatives, and doses are often reduced to allow for the increased sensitivity.

Natural Approaches

Acupressure/Tapping Considerations
Auricular Points
-NADA Protocol: Sympathetic, Shenmen, Liver, Kidney, Lung/Heart

Smoking: Sweetbreath – Midway between LU-7 and LI-5

Somatic Considerations
-Stress management and relaxation techniques such as visualization and meditation
-Counseling and support groups
-Regular exercise - at least 30 minutes 3 times per week, ex: brisk walking, aerobics, swimming, etc.
-Saunas and steam baths

Orthomolecular Considerations
- A multivitamin can be taken daily
-Glutamine – 500 to 1,000 milligrams 4 times per day between meals: to reduce craving for nicotine and other drugs.
-B-complex vitamins – 25 to 50 milligrams a day: Help reduce stress and tiredness.
-Vitamin C – 1,000 milligrams, 4 times a day for a week. Then take 1,000 milligrams twice a day

Phytotherapeutic Considerations
Alcohol:
-Oats: nervine, helps overcome habit
-Cayenne: delirium tremens; steadies patient, promotes sound sleep
-Chamomile: sedative
-White Fringetree: gastrointestinal or hepatic disorders
-Hops: delirium tremens, excitement, aids digestion
-Goldenseal: helps to overcome cravings
-Passionflower: insomnia; sedative
-Skullcap: delirium tremens, nervine: insomnia, nightmares, restlessness
-American Ginseng

Drug withdrawal:
-Oats: helps overcome habit (alcohol, morphine, opium)
-Chamomile: sedative
-Panax ginseng
-Skullcap: muscle twitchings

Smoking:
-Lobelia: aids withdrawal symptoms (stimulates nicotinergic receptors), expectorant
-Licorice Root: irritations of mucosa
-Milk Thistle: to clear toxins
-Valerian: to reduce anxiety and irritability and to aid in relaxation.
-Sweetflag: nerve tonic, helps overcome habit
-Fennel: helps expel mucous secretions
-Catnip: nervous irritability
-Passionflower: nervine, insomnia
-Bitter-berry (Chokeberry): sedative, quiets irritation of mucosa
-Skullcap: nervine
-Kola-nut: depressive states, melancholia
-Coltsfoot: to substitute habit

Dietary Considerations:
Alcohol withdrawal:
Eating principles:
-Once stabilized, a short alkaline fast is recommended, highly supervised. Good dietary habits are a must.

Therapeutic foods:
-Beets and beet tops, bamboo shoots, spinach, banana, grapefruit, mulberry, persimmon, strawberry, white mushroom, apple, ginseng, white fungus
-Daikon radish, pear, mandarin orange, black soybeans, dandelion, burdock, chlorophyll,

artichokes, garlic, onions
-Increase Zinc-rich foods, Magnesium-rich foods, foods with Vitamins B1 and B6; in beginning detoxification, supply with enough fruit juices to get lift when needed and enough liquid
-Dandelion tea

Avoid:
-Cinnamon and other heating foods, spicy foods, coffee (long term), sweets and sugary foods, high fat diet, fried foods, candies, simple carbohydrates, fatty foods, rich foods, chocolate, nuts, smoking, stress, constipation, hot foods, chili

Smoking and drug detoxification:
-All alcohol detoxification applies and fasting is recommended - increase all foods rich in vitamin A
- An alkalinizing diet to reduce nicotine cravings is recommended

Lifestyle and Additional Recommendations
-Create a deadline and decide on the date one begins to quit. This should be a time when there is minimal life stress and strain

-Establish a new routine. Changing one's routine will help break up old habit patterns that are associated with substance use.

-Fill the time that used to be spent using a substance with other activities and associations. Examples may include hobbies, starting a diary, reading, sewing, gardening, remodeling, learning a new skill or craft, creative arts activities, listening to music, taking music lessons, joining clubs, taking classes, or other social activities.

-If any of the withdrawal symptoms are causing extreme discomfort or seem to be getting worse even though several days have passed since you starting to quit, consider a medical examination.

-Nicotine: Quitting all at once has been shown to be a more successful strategy than just tapering down usage. Without cigarettes, the nicotine will clear out of the body in about 48 hours. This will help diminish cravings and give the body systems a chance to heal. Lobelia can be very helpful during this detoxification stage.

Appendix A:
Brodmann's Areas

Functions and Locations of Brodmann's Areas			
Brodmann Area	**Functional Area**	**Location**	**Function**
1, 2, 3	Primary somatic sensory cortex	Postcentral Gyrus	Touch
4	Primary motor cortex	Precentral Gyrus	Voluntary movement control
5	Tertiary somatic sensory cortex	Superior Parietal Lobule	Stereognosis
6	Premotor and supplementary motor	Precentral Gyrus	Limb and eye movement planning
7	Posterior parietal association area	Superior parietal lobule	Multimodal area for spatial body sense
8	Frontal eye lids	Posterio superior, middle frontal gyri	Saccadic eye movements
9, 10, 11, 12	Prefrontal association cortex	Superior, middle frontal gyri	Thought, cognition, ethics, moral, movement, planning
13, 14, 15, 16	Part of the insular cortex		
17	Primary visual cortex	Banks of calcarine tissue	Vision
18	Secondary visual cortex	Medial and lateral occipital gyri	Vision, depth
19	Tertiary visual cortex	Medial and lateral occipital gyri	Vision, color, motion, depth
20, 21	Visual inferotemporal area	Middle and inferior temporal gyrus	Form vision
22	Higher order auditory cortex	Superior temporal gyrus	Hearing, speech
23, 24, 25, 26, 27	Limbic association cortex	Cingulate gyrus, subcallosal area, parahippocampal gyrus	Emotions, attention, detection of error, novelty
28	Olfactory & Limbic cortex, sensoty multi-modal association	Parahippocampal gyrus	Smell, emotions, memory

	cortex		
29, 30, 31, 32, 33	Limbic association cortex	Cingulate gyrus	Emotions
34, 35, 36	Olfactory cortex & limbic cortex	Parahippocampal gyrus	Smell, emotions
37	Occipital association cortex	Middle and inferior temporal gyri	Perception, vision, reading, speech, movement
38	Olfactory & limbic cortex	Temporal pole	Smell, emotions, language
39	Parietal-association cortex	Inferior parietal lobule (angular gyrus)	Perception, vision, reading, speech
40	Parietal-temporal occipital association cortex	Inferior parietal lobule (supramarginal gyrus)	Reading, speech, movement
41, 42	Primary & Secondary auditory cortex	Heschyl's gyri & superior temporal gyrus	Hearing
43	Gustatory cortex	Insular cortex, frontoparietal operculum	Taste, GI tract
44, 45	Lateral premotor cortex (dominant hemisphere)	Inferior frontal gyrus (frontal operculum)	Speech, movement, planning
45	Prefrontal association cortex	Inferior frontal gyrus (frontal operculum)	Thought, cognition, planning, behavior
46	Dorsolateral prefrontal cortex	Middle frontal gyrus	Thought, cognition, plan, behavior, eye movement
47	Prefrontal association cortex	Inferior frontal gyus (frontal operculum)	Semantic speech area

REFERENCES

General References

Beck, Randy. *Functional Neurology For Practitioners of Manual Medicine.* Churchill Livingston. 2011. Print

Bercell, David. *The Revolutionary Trauma Release Process: transcend your toughest times.* Vancouver, Canada: Namaste Publishing. 2008 Print

Chen, John & Chen, Tina. *Chinese Herbal Formulas and Applications: pharmacological effects & clinical research.* City of Industry, CA: Art of Medicine Press. 2009. Print.

Chen, John, Chen, Tina., & Crampton, Laraine. *Chinese Medical Herbology and Pharmacology.* City of Industry, CA: Art of Medicine Press. 2004. Print.

Edward, Leon & Khan, Anum. *Concussion, Traumatic Brain Injury, mTBI: The ultimate TBI rehabilitation guide.* 2019. Print

Flaws, Bob & Lake, James. *Chinese Medical Psychiatry: a textbook and clinical manual: including indications for referral to Western medical services.* Boulder, CO: Blue Poppy. 2003. Print.

Joseph, R. *Neuropsychiatry, Neuropsychology and Clinical Neuroscience: emotion, evolution, cognition, language, memory, brain damage, and abnormal behavior.* Baltimore: Williams and Wilkins. 1996. Print

Kastner, Joerg. *Chinese Nutrition Therapy: dietetics in traditional Chinese medicine. 2nd Ed. New York*: Thieme. 2009. Print

Lash, Marilyn. *The Essential Brain Injury Guide.* 5th ed. Vienna, VA: Academy of Certified Brain Injury Specialists, Brain Injury Association of America. 2016. Print.

Marz, Russell. *Medical Nutrition From Marz: a textbook in clinical nutrition.* Portland, Or.: Omni-Press. 1999. Print.

Maciocia, Giovanni. *The Psyche in Chinese Medicine: treatment of emotional and mental disharmonies with acupuncture and Chinese herbs.* Churchill Livingstone. 2009. Print.

Morgan, Cara. *Concussion and Traumatic Brain Injury: a Chinese medical approach.* Portland, OR: National College of Naturopathic Medicine. 2005. Print.

Pizzorno, Joseph E. , Murray, Michael T. , & Joiner-Bey, Herb. *The Clinician's Handbook of Natural Medicine 2nd Ed*. St. Louis, Missouri: Churchill Livingstone Elsevier. 2008. Print

Prasah, Ph.D, Kedar. *Treat Concussion, TBI, and PTSD with Vitamins and Antioxidants*. Toronto, Canada: Healing Arts Press. 2016. Print

Silver, Jonathan, Yudofsky, Stuart, McAllister, Thomas. *Textbook of Traumatic Brain Injury*. Washington, DC: American Psychiatric Pub. 2011. Print.

Solie De Morant, George & Zmiewski, Paul. *Chinese Acupuncture*. Brookline, MA, U.S.A.: Paradigm Publications. 1994. Print.

Ward, Jamie. *The Students Guide to Cognitive Neuroscience*. London: Taylor and Francis. 2015. Print.

Wingate, Douglas S. *Healing Brain Injury with Chinese Medical Approaches*. London: Singing Dragon Publishing. 2018. Print.

Yang, Joseph. *Shen Disturbance: a guideline for psychiatry in traditional Chinese medicine*. Los Angeles. 2005. Print.

Zasler, Nathan, Katz, Douglas, & Zafonte, Ross. *Brain Injury Medicine: principles and practice*. New York, NY: Demos Medical Pub. 2013. Print.

NOTES:

NOTES: